# Tools for Building Culturally Competent HIV Prevention Programs

## with CD-ROM

**Josefina J. Card, PhD,** is Founder, President, and CEO of Sociometrics Corporation, an applied social science research and development (R&D) company based in Los Altos, CA. Dr. Card is a nationally recognized social scientist and an expert in the establishment and operation of research-based social science resources, products and services. She has served as Principal Investigator of over 70 research-to-practice R&D projects, most of them funded by the U.S. National Institutes of Health. These R&D projects have resulted in the development of several hundred social science–based commercial products, including the exemplary data sets, effective intervention programs, and evaluation and training materials comprising the Social Science Electronic Data Library; the Program Archive on Sexuality, Health & Adolescence; the HIV/AIDS Prevention Program Archive; and the Institute for Program Development and Evaluation. These resources have been used by thousands of academic as well as health practitioner customers in schools, clinics and communities across the country. Alongside her track record as a project manager, Dr. Card has established a solid track record as a health and population scientist. She has authored over 80 books, monographs, and journal articles. Her work is noted for its integration of behavioral, social, psychological, and demographic perspectives. Throughout her career, Dr. Card has recognized the importance of communicating scientific findings both to scientists as well as to other professionals (service providers, policy makers, health practitioners) and lay citizens who could benefit from the body of knowledge. Dr. Card has also devoted a significant portion of her career to facilitating the development and scientific evaluation of social intervention programs. She has served as a member of many federal advisory committees, including the NIH (National Institutes of Health) Study Section for Social Sciences and Population, the NICHD (National Institute on Child Health and Human Development) Population Research Committee, and the NICHD Advisory Council. Dr. Card is also active in the community. While her children were in school she served as PTA officer, founded the Gunn High School Parent Community Service Boosters, and chaired the Gunn Parent-Teacher Wish List Fund. She also served as Chair of the Palo Alto Unified School District Housing Options for Teachers project, aimed at bringing and keeping outstanding teachers in the award-winning PAUSD school district. From 1999 to 2003 she worked with the Packard Foundation, the Santa Clara County Public Health Department, and the Adolescent Pregnancy Prevention Network in an effort that lowered the County's teen pregnancy and birth rates by over 40%, surpassing the also-impressive performances by the State and nation in this regard. Currently Dr. Card, a native of the Philippines, is working with Pathways Philippines and with the Ayala Foundation USA to raise funds to allow outstanding graduates of Philippine public high schools to go to college.

**Julie Solomon, PhD,** serves as a Senior Research Associate and the Director of Training Support at Sociometrics Corporation. As a Senior Research Associate, she has directed R&D, evaluation, and consulting projects in diverse behavioral health areas, including HIV, STI, and teen pregnancy prevention; substance abuse prevention; violence prevention; and clinician-patient communication in the context of (patient) communication disorders. These projects have been funded by a variety of public and private entities, including the National Institutes of Health (NIH), the David & Lucile Packard Foundation, Johnson & Johnson Corporate Contributions, the California Healthy Kids Resource Center, and the Santa Clara County (California) Public Health Department. As Director of Training Support at Sociometrics, Dr. Solomon develops and delivers workshops on program planning and evaluation for diverse audiences, principally practitioners in the sexual and reproductive health fields. Dr. Solomon joined Sociometrics in 1999 after completing a PhD in linguistics at Stanford University. While in graduate school, she taught in several departments and also worked for ETR Associates, the American Institutes for Research (AIR), and the Palo Alto Medical Foundation Research Institute on projects addressing sexual behavior and HIV risk among Latino youth and adults in California. A common thread that runs through much of Dr. Solomon's work is a desire to empower health and social service providers to carry out appropriate cultural adaptation and successful replication of empirically validated prevention programs. She has recently published on these topics through the National Campaign to Prevent Teen Pregnancy and in the journal *Evaluation and the Health Professions.* In addition to coauthoring *The Complete HIV/AIDS Teaching Kit with CD-ROM,* she is also a coauthor of *Tools for Building Culturally Competent HIV Prevention Programs* (Springer Publishing Company, 2007).

**Jacqueline Berman, PhD,** cowrote this book while she was a Senior Research Associate at Sociometrics Corporation. Dr. Berman is currently a Principal Analyst with Berkeley Policy Associates. She has directed a number of social policy projects in the areas of international human rights, welfare reform, educational advancement, HIV, STI and teen pregnancy prevention, gender mainstreaming, youth violence prevention, cultural difference, and disaster relief for the U.S. Departments of Labor, Education, and State, various state and city governments, and a number of private foundations. A former professor of international relations, Dr. Berman has conducted extensive field research in eastern, southeastern, and western Europe on issues related to human rights, human security, violence prevention, and gender justice. Her research has been supported by the Fulbright Program, the Woodrow Wilson Foundation, the Social Science Research Council, the MacArthur Foundation, and the Rockefeller Foundation. She has published on a number of topics including human security, human rights, violence prevention, reproductive health, education programs, welfare reform, cultural practices, and gender rights.

# Tools for Building Culturally Competent HIV Prevention Programs

with **CD-ROM**

**AUTHORS** Josefina J. Card
Julie Solomon
Jacqueline Berman

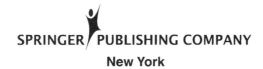

SPRINGER PUBLISHING COMPANY

**New York**

Springer Publishing Company, LLC
11 West 42nd Street
New York, NY 10036
www.springerpub.com

*Acquisitions Editor: Jennifer Perillo*
*Production Editor: Shana Meyer*
*Cover design: Joanne E. Honigman*
*Composition: Aptara Inc.*

08  09  10  11/5  4  3  2  1

---

**Library of Congress Cataloging-in-Publication Data**

Card, Josefina J.
   Tools for building culturally competent HIV prevention programs / Josefina J. Card, Julie Solomon, Jacqueline Berman.
        p.  ;  cm.
   Includes bibliographical references and index.
   ISBN 978-0-8261-1517-1 (softcover)
  1. AIDS (Disease)—United States—Prevention—Cross-cultural studies.   2. HIV infections—United States—Prevention—Cross-cultural studies.   3. AIDS (Disease)—Study and teaching—United States.   4. HIV infections—Study and teaching—United States.   5. Transcultural medical care—United States.   I. Solomon, Julie, 1968–
II. Berman, Jacqueline.   III. Title.
   [DNLM: 1. HIV Infections—prevention & control.   2. Cultural Diversity.   3. Ethnic Groups—psychology.   4. Health Education—methods.   5. Minority Groups—psychology.   6. United States. WC 503.6 C266t 2008]
RA643.5.C37   2008
362.196′9792—dc22

2007030108

---

Printed in the United States of America by Bang Printing

# Acknowledgments

The authors wish to thank Angela Amarillas, Megan Bunch, Diana Dull Akers, and Patricia Vinh-Thomas, who developed some of the cultural competence-related concepts, tales, and tools in this book; Laura Lessard, who provided outstanding editorial assistance; Tamara Kuhn and Ruben Ruiz, who produced the associated Web site and CD-ROM; and the National Institute of Allergy and Infectious Diseases (NIAID) of the National Institutes of Health (NIH), which provided funding for the effort.

# Dedication

For Stu, Adam, and Jaimey

# Contents

In the absence of a vaccine, behavioral prevention is still the best tool available for stemming the tide of HIV infection (Stryker et al., 1995). Research has shown strong evidence for the effectiveness of behavioral interventions in changing HIV-related risk behaviors and reducing the incidence of HIV infection among vulnerable populations, including populations that historically have proven difficult to reach (Card et al., 2001; Crepaz et al., 2006; Lyles et al., 2007).

Recent literature on racial disparities in HIV/AIDS and effective HIV/AIDS prevention programs underscores the importance of cultural sensitivity, cultural relevance, and cultural competence in the delivery of services and care (Auerbach & Coates, 2000; Bok & Morales, 2001; Scott et al., 2005; Vinh-Thomas et al., 2003; Wilson & Miller, 2003). HIV risk behaviors are heavily influenced by underlying socioeconomic conditions (such as poverty, discrimination, and underemployment) as well as cultural norms (in terms of gender, sexuality, health, and illness). Therefore, successful prevention interventions must be tailored for their target populations, address the multiple factors influencing individual risk, and pay special attention to the sociocultural factors that influence behavior (Hernandez & Smith, 1991; Zenilman et al., 2001).

The need for cultural competence in the delivery of health services has long been recognized by practitioners, researchers, and funding agencies. In recent years, a growing literature on the importance of attaining cultural competence and on the various conceptualizations of cultural competence has emerged, reflecting the increasingly prominent role that the concept now plays in discussions among researchers and practitioners, particularly as they relate to reducing racial disparities (Brach & Fraser, 2000; Giger et al., 2007; Shaya & Gbarayor, 2006; Zembrana et al., 2004). Numerous social, public health, and medical service organizations have articulated their respective definitions of cultural competence. The U.S. Department of Health and Human Services convened a national advisory committee to propose Recommended Standards for Culturally and Linguistically Appropriate Health Care Services. The proposed standards were intended to promote a common understanding of cultural and linguistic competence in order to, among other things, eliminate racial and ethnic disparities (OMH, 2001).

Yet, despite the considerable emphasis on cultural competence, there is no widely accepted, functional definition of cultural competence that is specifically relevant to prevention. Not only does this mean that researchers have been unable to quantify cultural competence in order to rigorously test the relationship between cultural competence and prevention program effectiveness, but it also means that any program wishing to provide culturally competent HIV/AIDS prevention faces both a puzzling array of definitions, and no clear way to operationalize the concepts in practice.

This book is designed to elucidate the concepts of culture and cultural competence. Beyond this, it is aimed at helping HIV prevention professionals who are planning, implementing, or evaluating programs to increase the cultural competence and effectiveness of HIV prevention efforts in their local communities.

Section 1 introduces the notions of culture and cultural competence and discusses their link to HIV risk and HIV prevention. Sections 2–4 address HIV prevention program planning, implementation, and evaluation, respectively. Each of these latter three chapters:

- Summarizes in plain language the important research-based concepts and practices in effective, culturally competent HIV prevention programming.
- Exemplifies—through a series of "tales from the field"—how these key research-based principles and methods have been put into practice in real-world prevention settings.
- Offers user-friendly tools, including checklists and worksheets that facilitate culturally competent programming.

A CD-ROM accompanying the book provides electronic versions of the tools in Microsoft Word format. This allows the user to customize, print, and save each document for future use. The CD-ROM also includes a demo of the Virtual Program Evaluation Consultant (VPEC), a program evaluation software tool offered by Sociometrics. Purchasers of this book will get a three-month license to VPEC free.

A glossary of all terms used in the book is included at the end.

The book's content and features were informed by the scientific literature in HIV prevention and related fields, by Federal standards and guidelines for health care and social service provision, as well as by needs assessment research, usability testing, and field testing in collaboration with HIV prevention professionals working in diverse cultural contexts.

We hope that those working at the frontline to prevent HIV/AIDS and its risky behavior antecedents will find this book helpful to their work.

## REFERENCES

Auerbach, J. D., & Coates, T. J. (2000). Commentaries—HIV prevention research: Accomplishments and challenges for the third decade of AIDS. *American Journal of Public Health, 90*(7), 1029–1032.

Bok, M., & Morales, J. (2001). Latino communities in the U.S. and HIV/AIDS. *Journal of HIV/AIDS Prevention and Education for Adolescents and Children, 4*(1), 61–70.

Brach, C., & Fraser, I. (2000). Can cultural competency reduce racial and ethnic health disparities? A review and conceptual model. *Medical Care Research and Review, 57*(Suppl 1), 181–217.

Card, J. J., Benner, T., Shields, J. P., & Feinstein, N. (2001). The HIV/AIDS Prevention Program Archive (HAPPA): A collection of promising prevention programs in a box. *AIDS Education and Prevention, (13)*1, 1–28.

Crepaz, N., Lyles, C. M., Wolitski, R. J., Passin, W. F., Rama, S. M., Herbst, J. H., et al., & the HIV Prevention Research Synthesis (PRS) Team. (2006). Do prevention interventions reduce HIV risk behaviours among people living with HIV? A meta-analytic review of controlled trials. *AIDS, 20*(2), 143–157.

Giger, J., Davidhizar, R. E., Purnell, L., Harden, J. T., Phillips, J., Strickland, O., & American Academy of Nursing. (2007). American Academy of Nursing Expert Panel report: Developing cultural competence to eliminate health disparities in ethnic minorities and other vulnerable populations. *Journal of Transcultural Nursing, 18*(2), 95–102.

Hernandez, J. T., & Smith, F. J. (1991). Racial targeting of AIDS programs reconsidered. *Journal of the National Medical Association, 83*(1), 17–21.

Lyles, C. M., Kay, L. S., Crepaz, N., Herbst, J. H., Passin, W. F., Kim, A. S., et al., & the HIV/AIDS Prevention Research Synthesis Team. (2007). Best-evidence interventions: Findings from a systematic review of HIV behavioral interventions for US populations at high risk, 2000–2004. *American Journal of Public Health, 97*(1), 133–143.

Office of Minority Health (OMH), U.S. Department of Health and Human Services. (2001). *National standards for culturally and linguistically appropriate services in health care: Final report.* Washington, DC: OMH. Retrieved January 16, 2006, from http://www.omhrc.gov/assets/pdf/checked/finalreport.pdf

Scott, K. D., Gilliam, A., & Braxton, K. (2005). Culturally competent HIV prevention strategies for women of color in the United States. *Health Care for Women International, 26*(1), 17–45.

Shaya, F. T., & Gbarayor, C. M. (2006). The case for cultural competence in health professions education. *American Journal of Pharmaceutical Education, 70*(6), 124.

Stryker, J., Coates, T. J., DeCarlo, P., Haynes-Sanstad, K., Shriver, M., & Makadon, H. J. (1995). Prevention of HIV infection: Looking back, looking ahead. *The Journal of the American Medical Association, 273*(14), 1143–1148.

Vinh-Thomas, P., Bunch, M. M., & Card, J. J. (2003). A research-based tool for identifying and strengthening culturally competent and evaluation-ready HIV/AIDS prevention programs. *AIDS Education and Prevention, 15*(6), 481–498.

Wilson, B. D. M., & Miller, R. L. (2003). Examining strategies for culturally grounded HIV prevention: A review. *AIDS Education and Prevention, 15*(2), 184–202.

Zambrana, R. E., Molnar, C., Munoz, H. B., & Lopez, D. S. (2004). Cultural competency as it intersects with racial/ethnic. Linguistic, and class disparities in managed healthcare organizations. *The American Journal of Managed Care, 10*(Spec. No.), SP37-SP44.

Zenilman, J. M., Shahmanesh, M., & Winter, A. J. (2001). Ethnicity and STIs: More than black and white. *Sexually Transmitted Infections, 77*(1), 2–3.

# List of Tools

# Tools for Building Culturally Competent HIV Prevention Programs

# Introduction: What Is Culture?

## DEFINING CULTURE

When we think about *culture*, we often think about things like foods and festivals, or costumes and customs. But cultures are more than just collections of objects and practices (although these are aspects of culture). Most definitions of culture include the following elements (Brown, 1991; Scheer, 1994; Wilson & Miller, 2003):

- Culture comprises a widely shared set of values, institutions, practices, and beliefs that emerge—and change—as a group adapts to its environment.
- Culture is learned through social interactions that provide contexts for behavior and influence behavior.
- Cultural traditions are passed down through generations.

## A Person Combines Many Cultural Backgrounds

People never have just one cultural background. Instead, people come from and interact with a wide variety of cultures. Common examples of cultural categories include *race* and *ethnicity,* such as Asian American, White, Arab, Latino, African American, or Native American; *national origin,* such as French, Japanese, Moroccan, or Peruvian; and *religion,* such as Christian, Jewish, Moslem, or Hindu. Social class, immigration status, sexual orientation, gender, and age can also be considered cultural categories, because each such affiliation (e.g., working or upper class, undocumented or second generation, gay or straight, female or transgender, teen or senior citizen) is associated with a common set of values, norms, and practices. Groups with common interests, such as runners, punk-rockers, or injection drug users, and group with common experiences, such as HIV-seropositive people, survivors of sexual abuse, veterans, and persons with physical disabilities, can be considered cultural groups for the same reason. Persons from the same geographic region (e.g., New Englanders, Southerners), political orientation (right-wing or left-wing), or age cohort (e.g., Generation X) can also share a cultural background.

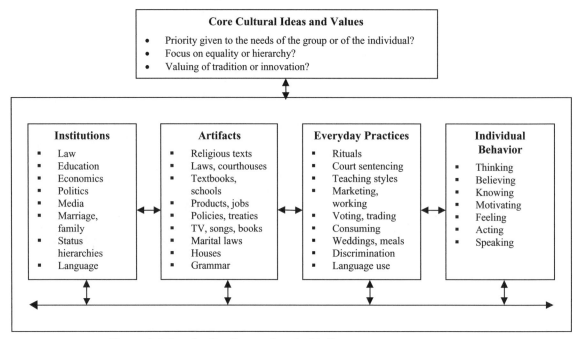

**Figure 1-1  Levels of culture and mutual influences.**

Because of the many cultural categories, cultural identity varies within both groups and individuals. For example, "Asian American" is an extremely broad term that can refer to both second-generation Buddhist Vietnamese Americans and recent Moslem immigrants from Pakistan. These groups hold extremely different cultural beliefs and practices. At the same time, each person within a group has a different sense of themselves in relation to their cultural identities. For example, an individual may identify more strongly with being lesbian than with being Asian American or a second-generation immigrant. HIV prevention programming needs to take into account diversity both across and within clients' cultural groups, as well as the multiple cultural identities of individuals in those groups.

## WHERE DOES CULTURE COME FROM?

### Individuals and Cultures Shape Each Other

People are shaped by the cultures with which they interact. By thinking, feeling, and acting according to their cultures, individuals reproduce their cultures. In this way, cultures and people shape each other.

In brief, each cultural group has a set of core ideas and values. For example, some cultures emphasize the needs of the group over the needs or desires of any individual in the group. Other cultures place greater emphasis on self-reliance and personal independence. Core ideas and values such as these shape the culture's institutions, objects, and everyday activities, as well as the behavior of individual group members. But the institutions, objects, practices, and behaviors also influence each other—and they constantly shape and reshape the core ideas and values of the group. Figure 1–1 illustrates this process.

### Learning and Teaching Culture

When children are born, or when people arrive to a new culture, they are generally not given a rulebook or a lecture on how to be a culturally appropriate person. Instead, they learn many of the culture's core ideas and values implicitly from that culture's institutions, artifacts, and practices as well as from family and other primary social groups, such as friends, acquaintances, and coworkers. For example, young children learn cultural values by watching older members of their household and community. By thinking, feeling, and acting according to the culture's blueprints, the new cultural members rebuild the culture for others. Most of the time, people don't think about themselves as producers and reproducers of culture. Rather, they think they are just having a conversation, cooking dinner, or putting their children to bed like any other normal person would. People cannot remember when they learned many of the basic rules of their culture, and unless they are immersed in different cultures, they may not even realize that their ways of thinking, feeling, and acting are different from those of other cultural groups.

As a prevention practitioner, you can take steps to be more aware of the similarities and differences between your own cultural values and beliefs and those of your program participants. This is a key step in learning to work more effectively with clients of diverse backgrounds.

## WHAT DOES CULTURE HAVE TO DO WITH HIV?

### The Impact of HIV/AIDS on Different Populations in the United States

In the United States, people in some cultural groups or communities become infected with HIV and develop AIDS at higher rates than people in others. For example:

- In 2005, rates of HIV/AIDS cases in the United States were 72.8 per 100,000 in the Black population, 28.5 per 100,000 in the Hispanic population, 10.6 per 100,000 in the American Indian/Alaska Native population, 9.0 in the White population, and 7.6 per 100,000 in the Asian/Pacific Islander population (Centers for Disease Control and Prevention [CDC], 2006).
- According to a study of U.S. Job Corps applicants, HIV prevalence among African-American adolescent girls was 4.9 per 1,000, whereas rates among white and Hispanic adolescent girls were 0.7 and 0.6. Similarly, rates among white, Hispanic, and African-American adolescent boys were 0.8, 1.5, and 3.2 (respectively) per 1,000 (Valleroy et al., 1998).
- From 2001 through 2005, the estimated number of HIV/AIDS cases in the U.S. increased among men who have sex with men (MSM). MSM accounted for 49% of all HIV/AIDS cases diagnosed in 2005 (CDC, 2006).

As these statistics suggest, HIV and AIDS have a differential impact on diverse cultural groups.

### Links Between HIV/AIDS and Culture

The trends in HIV/AIDS risk and infection are not limited to the United States. Researchers Raj, Amaro, and Reed have completed global analyses of those most impacted by HIV/AIDS and found that while these groups are diverse, they share commonalties: "They are marginalized within their societies . . . [and are] oppressed because of race, class, gender, or non-conformity to socially prescribed behaviors . . . " (Raj, Amaro, & Reed, 2001, p. 196). For example (Joint U.N. Programme [UNAIDS]/WHO, 2006):

- In sub-Saharan Africa in 2006, 59% of the HIV-positive (HIV+) adult population was female. In many Asian, Eastern European, and Latin American countries, the proportions of HIV+ women continue to grow.

RACISM: Hispanic gay men who reported more risky sex also reported having experienced more racism as children and adults (Diaz et al., 2000; Marín, 2003).

POVERTY: *Jornaleros* (day workers) may be sexually exploited by employers or forced to sell sex to support themselves and their families (Marín, 2003).

HOMOPHOBIA: Hispanic gay men who experience greater levels of homophobia report more sexual risk behavior (Diaz, 1998; Marín, 2003).

TRADITIONAL GENDER ROLES: To prove "manhood," Hispanic men may seek many sexual partners. Hispanic women may sometimes feel unable to insist on safer sex practices, such as condom use, with male partners (Gómez & Marín, 1996; Marín, 2003; Marín et al., 1993).

ACCULTURATION: Less acculturated Hispanic middle school youth have less knowledge about HIV/AIDS than their more acculturated peers. The less acculturated girls are less sexually active, but they also have less confidence in condom effectiveness. The less acculturated boys are more sexually active at earlier ages (Marsiglia & Navarro, 1999).

HEALTH CARE: Hispanics typically seek HIV/AIDS treatment late in the course of the disease. They face limited access to health care, because of factors such as lack of insurance and language barriers, as well as withholding of highly active antiretroviral therapy (HAART) by care providers (Butcher et al., 2005; Santos et al., 2004).

**Figure 1-2  An example of social, cultural, and economic influences on HIV risk: Hispanics in the United States.**

- In Central and Eastern Europe in 2005, 67% of HIV+ persons had acquired HIV through use of nonsterile injection drug use equipment.
- In South and Southeast Asia (excluding India) in 2005, 8% of HIV+ persons were commercial sex workers and 41% of HIV+ persons were their clients.
- HIV outbreaks among men who have sex with men are on the rise in a number of Asian countries, including Cambodia, China, India, Nepal, Pakistan, Thailand, and Vietnam. In very few of these countries do national AIDS programs adequately address risk among MSM.

Disparities in HIV rates (and other health-related conditions) are linked to broad, underlying social, cultural, and economic issues, such as poverty, racism and discrimination, sexism, violence, and inadequate health care systems. In addition, culture shapes attitudes and beliefs that in turn influence individuals' HIV/AIDS-related risk and protective behaviors. For example, culture shapes definitions of health and illness, beliefs about what causes disease and how to prevent it, attitudes toward communicating about HIV-related behaviors, and attitudes toward changing HIV-related behaviors. Culture can also affect the ability of providers and clients to communicate effectively and clients' comfort in using services. An example of how diverse social, cultural, and economic factors influence HIV/AIDS risk among U.S. Hispanics is provided in Figure 1–2.

## WHAT IS CULTURAL COMPETENCE?

### Our Definition of Cultural Competence

*Cultural competence* has been defined somewhat differently by diverse fields of research and practice. In this book, we follow researchers Vinh-Thomas, Bunch, and Card (2003) in defining it as:

A set of congruent behaviors, attitudes, and policies—including a consideration of linguistic, socioeconomic, and functional concerns that influence behavior (like et al., 1996)—that come together in a system, agency, or among professionals, thus:

*Standards Concerning Culturally Competent Care*

**Standard 1.** Health care organizations should ensure that patients/consumers receive from all staff members effective, understandable, and respectful care that is provided in a manner compatible with their cultural health beliefs and practices and preferred language.

**Standard 2.** Health care organizations should implement strategies to recruit, retain, and promote at all levels of the organization a diverse staff and leadership that are representative of the demographic characteristics of the service area.

**Standard 3.** Health care organizations should ensure that staff at all levels and across all disciplines receive ongoing education and training in culturally and linguistically appropriate service delivery.

*Standards Concerning Language Access Services*

**Standard 4.** Health care organizations must offer and provide language assistance services, including bilingual staff and interpreter services, at no cost to each patient/consumer with limited English proficiency at all points of contact, in a timely manner during all hours of operation.

**Standard 5.** Health care organizations must provide to patients/consumers in their preferred language both verbal offers and written notices informing them of their right to receive language assistance services.

**Standard 6.** Health care organizations must assure the competence of language assistance provided to limited English proficient patients/consumers by interpreters and bilingual staff. Family and friends should not be used to provide interpretation services (except on request by the patient/consumer).

**Standard 7.** Health care organizations must make available easily understood patient-related materials and post signage in the languages of the commonly encountered groups and/or groups represented in the service area.

*Standards Concerning Organizational Supports for Cultural Competence*

**Standard 8.** Health care organizations should develop, implement, and promote a written strategic plan that outlines clear goals, policies, operational plans, and management accountability/oversight mechanisms to provide culturally and linguistically appropriate services.

**Standard 9.** Health care organizations should conduct initial and ongoing organizational self-assessments of CLAS-related activities and are encouraged to integrate cultural and linguistic competence-related measures into their internal audits, performance improvement programs, patient satisfaction assessments, and outcomes-based evaluations.

**Standard 10.** Health care organizations should ensure that data on the individual patient's/consumer's race, ethnicity, and spoken and written language are collected in health records, integrated into the organization's management information systems, and periodically updated.

**Standard 11.** Health care organizations should maintain a current demographic, cultural, and epidemiological profile of the community as well as a needs assessment to accurately plan for and implement services that respond to the cultural and linguistic characteristics of the service area.

**Standard 12.** Health care organizations should develop participatory, collaborative partnerships with communities and utilize a variety of formal and informal mechanisms to facilitate community and patient/consumer involvement in designing and implementing CLAS-related activities.

**Standard 13.** Health care organizations should ensure that conflict and grievance resolution processes are culturally and linguistically sensitive and capable of identifying, preventing, and resolving cross-cultural conflicts or complaints by patients/consumers.

**Standard 14.** Health care organizations are encouraged to regularly make available to the public information about their progress and successful innovations in implementing the CLAS standards and to provide public notice in their communities about the availability of this information.

**Figure 1-3  National Standards for Culturally and Linguistically Appropriate Services (CLAS) in Health Care (OMH, 2001, pp. 7–20).**

Field-Specific Definitions of Cultural Competence

| Medicine | Cultural competence is a process that requires individual staff members and health care systems to develop and expand their ability to effectively know about, be sensitive to, and have respect for cultural diversity (Association of American Medical Colleges, 1998; Flores, 1997; Suh, 2004). |
|---|---|
| Psychology | Culturally competent psychotherapy comprises proper interpersonal communication and a relationship between psychologists and ethnically different patients. A culturally competent psychologist is aware of diversity and has the knowledge, communication skills, and attitudes necessary to provide effective care for diverse populations (Sue, 1998; Sue & Zane, 1987; Suh, 2004). |
| Education | Cultural competence in school education is composed of awareness and acceptance of cultural differences, awareness of the teacher's own cultural values, knowledge of the students' culture, and ability to adapt practical skills to fit the students' cultural context. It includes an ongoing process of growth through questioning, self-assessment, knowledge, and skill-building that starts with students' current competencies and supports expansion of their abilities (Grant & Haynes, 1995; McManus, 1988; Sowers-Hoag & Sandau-Beckler, 1996; Suh, 2004). |
| Social Work | Cultural competence is a process of striving to increase self-awareness, value diversity, and become knowledgeable about cultural strengths and vulnerabilities of families (Bonecutter & Gleeson, 1997; Suh, 2004). |
| Nursing | Cultural competence is the process in which the health care provider strives to achieve the capacity to work effectively within the client's cultural context (individual, family, or community) (Campinha-Bacote, 1994; Suh, 2004). |

(1) enabling that system, agency, or those professionals to work effectively with the target population (Cross et al., 1989) and

(2) resulting in services that are accepted by the target population (Dana et al., 1992).

## Federal Standards for Culturally Competent Health Care

In 1997, the U.S. Office of Minority Health (OMH) undertook development of a set of health care standards that embodied this conceptualization of cultural competence. The resultant 14 *National Standards for Culturally and Linguistically Appropriate Services in Health Care (CLAS)*, shown in Figure 1–3, are designed to provide clear guidance on culturally competent service provision to providers, policy makers, accreditation and credentialing agencies, patients, advocates, educators, and the health care community in general. The ultimate aim of the standards is to contribute to the elimination of racial and ethnic health disparities, such as HIV/AIDS incidence and prevalence, and to improve the health of all Americans (OMH, 2001).

## Other Definitions of Cultural Competence

Although many staff working in HIV prevention come from health-related disciplines, others come from social service or other backgrounds. Each field has traditionally defined and approached cultural competence in its own way. Examples of some discipline-specific definitions are provided in Table 1–1.

As you work to develop a definition of cultural competence for your agency or program (see Defining Your Terms), you may want to use one or more of the

- According to the 2000 U.S. Census, more than 30% of the population is composed of ethnic and racial minorities (Grieco, 2001).

- The number of persons identifying themselves as members of ethnic and racial minority groups is expected to grow to nearly 50% of the U.S. population by 2050 (Day, 1996).

- According to a 2005 household survey conducted by the U.S. Bureau of Labor Statistics (BLS), only 10% of Registered Nurses are African American, 6.4% are Asian, and 4.3% are Latino (BLS, 2006).

- Only about 6% of practicing physicians are Latino, African American, or Native American (American Medical Student Association, 2006).

**Figure 1-4  Diversity: A health care example.**

definitions provided here as a starting point for discussion. Ultimately, how you define cultural competence should reflect the unique needs and perspectives of your target population, agency, and community.

# WHAT DOES CULTURAL COMPETENCE HAVE TO DO WITH HIV PREVENTION?

## Different Cultures of Providers and Clients

HIV prevention program staff and their clients may be from different cultural backgrounds. As is exemplified in Figure 1–4, service providers are often college-educated, middle-class, and majority group members (e.g., white, English-speaking, heterosexual, not injection drug users, etc.), whereas program clients are often from more diverse backgrounds. Service providers and their clients often differ with respect to language, literacy level, access to resources, beliefs about health and illness, and health practices. As a result, those who develop, deliver, and assess HIV prevention programs may have difficulty understanding and addressing the needs of those served by the programs. Recent research has shown that interactions between caregivers and clients influence clients' care-seeking and level of participation in health-related services. Culturally competent providers can improve clients' care-seeking, increase their enrollment in research studies to assess HIV prevention and treatment regimens, and improve their adherence to HIV antiretroviral therapy (Butler et al., 2005; Lum, 2003; Scott et al., 2005; Schilder et al., 2001; Stevenson & White, 1994; Stone et al., 1998). It is therefore important that service agencies and providers strive to change their own knowledge, attitudes, skills, behaviors, and policies in ways that promote more effective communication with clients, improved access to services, and greater acceptance of those services.

## Cultural Influences on HIV Risk

Because culture is linked to HIV transmission, health and social service providers need to take culture into account when planning, implementing, and evaluating HIV prevention programs. In particular, current research suggests that to achieve positive intervention outcomes, it is important to recognize cultural, social, and economic factors that influence HIV risk and protective behaviors, as well as access to prevention and treatment services. These factors include broad societal-level forces (e.g., poverty, racism, sexism), as well as individual and community-based beliefs, attitudes, norms about gender roles, communication among sexual partners, and health and illness.

## BUILDING CULTURALLY COMPETENT PROGRAMS

### The Building Blocks of Cultural Competence

Building culturally competent HIV prevention programs involves addressing the culturally related needs of program participants. Doing this requires an ongoing process of:

- **Looking inward** at agency and staff norms, values, beliefs, and assumptions
- **Looking outward** at how cultural factors affect HIV-related behaviors and access to an use of services
- **Applying knowledge** to HIV prevention programming in ways that address cultural factors relevant to HIV prevention
- **Actively involving clients** in planning, implementation, and evaluation processes and treating them with respect and sensitivity

In particular, it is always a good idea to review relevant research reports and articles on populations that are similar to your clients, so that you do not waste time "reinventing the wheel" or using strategies that have already been shown not to work. It is also important to address the various cultural dimensions (e.g., gender, race/ethnicity, sexual orientation, immigration status, etc.) that have an impact on their risk behaviors and on their ability and inclination to access prevention services. Finally, it is essential to involve target population members in program planning, implementation, and evaluation activities in meaningful ways that make them feel part of—rather than marginalized by—HIV-related programming. Subsequent sections will help you to incorporate these and other essential cultural competence-related activities into your HIV prevention efforts.

### Cultural Competence at the Individual, Program, and Agency Levels

The principal focus of subsequent sections is culturally competent program planning, implementation, and evaluation. However, as was indicated earlier, culturally competent programming efforts are impacted by both individual staff members' attitudes and actions, as well as their agencies' policies and practices. For those interested in assessing cultural competence among individual staff members or agency-wide, a variety of tools are available from other sources—see the references at the end of this section.

## DEFINING YOUR TERMS

A crucial first step in building culturally competent programs is to develop or adapt a working definition of culture. Articulating this definition will help program planners, implementers, and evaluators to achieve a common understanding about what culture means in their local context, identify relevant cultural categories for local HIV prevention efforts, and address community-level cultural factors that are relevant for HIV prevention (Wilson & Miller, 2003).

A second important step in building culturally competent programs is to develop or adapt a working definition of cultural competence. This definition will help program staff and consultants to achieve a shared understanding what cultural competence means and involves and integrate cultural competence into program planning, implementation, and evaluation. It will also help program personnel explain to others what cultural competence is, why it is important, and how their program or program evaluation will address it.

*Project Street Beat,* an HIV outreach program of *Planned Parenthood of New York City, Inc.,* works with homeless and street populations of four New York City boroughs (the Bronx, Manhattan, Brooklyn, and Queens). The program defines culture broadly to include not only the race/ethnicity and language background of clients but also their age, gender, and sexuality. In addition, Project Street Beat considers the environmental, behavioral, and linguistic aspects of poverty, addiction, and street life in New York City as part of their definition of culture. For example, sex is the key currency in the drug economy of the New York City streets. Understanding the cultures of substance abuse and commercial sex work permits Project Street Beat to address their clients' HIV-related needs and service barriers through culturally appropriate HIV and medical outreach, education, crisis intervention, and referrals. The program uses former clients as peer outreach workers and provides them with mentoring and support to help them stay drug-free and address personal and on-the-job challenges (HRSA, 2001, pp. 12, 48).

*Betances Health Unit, Inc.,* is a community-based medical provider that serves the Latino population of Lower Manhattan, New York City. In the agency's view, cultural competence is demonstrated not only by broad knowledge of the cultural groups represented but also by practical experience with the communities served. In accordance with this view, the agency identifies two types of cultural competence. They define *indigenous cultural competence* as cultural knowledge that is the result of birth and life experience, and *acquired cultural competence* as acquired knowledge that reflects varying levels of language and sociocultural proficiency. Betances values both types and draws on a combination of these competencies within their staff to promote peer-to-peer dialogue, training, and problem-solving, in service of their clients' needs. Agency staff, who include both Latino and non-Latino providers, deliver a wide range of Western medical services, mental health and substance abuse counseling, and holistic treatments that are aligned with diverse, culture-specific practices. The program also conducts outreach to local Latino communities (HRSA, 2001, pp. 13, 50).

**Figure 1-5 Examples of definitions of culture and cultural competence from the Cultural Competence Works Competition (HRSA, 2001).**

To develop your own definitions of culture and cultural competence, it is helpful to:

1. Review existing definitions of culture and cultural competence, such as those in Table 1–1 and in Figure 1–5.
2. Meet with all key stakeholders (e.g., program staff, other agency staff, members of the local community) to discuss and reach agreement on your own definitions.
3. Write down the definitions and circulate them to key stakeholders for review and feedback.

The federal government's Health Resources and Services Administration (HRSA) sponsored a "Cultural Competence Works" competition in 1998 to recognize and honor outstanding HRSA-funded programs and highlight their culturally competent services (HRSA, 2001). HRSA found that nominated programs tended to define culture broadly and take into account how various cultural memberships and identities contribute to access to care, quality of care, and health outcomes. Nominated programs also tended to consider a cultural group's historical relationship with the medical establishment in seeking to provide appropriate services. Examples of these programs' perspectives on culture and cultural competence are provided in Figure 1–5.

Once you have developed your working definitions, make sure that they are publicized and used to the benefit of your programming efforts. To publicize the definitions, consider incorporating them into staff trainings and meetings. Post them for reference in your agency lunchroom, conference room, and client service areas. Include them in program materials, presentations, and reports that are disseminated to agency boards, community members, policy makers, and funders. Challenge program staff and managers to use the definitions to identify specific actions to be taken in program planning, implementation, or evaluation efforts. For example, you might ask yourself and your colleagues: How could the physical setting of service provision, client intake procedures, program materials, or evaluation surveys be made more culturally competent, as you have defined the term?

## REFERENCES

American Medical Student Association (AMSA). (2006). Diversity in medicine. Retrieved March 21, 2006, from http://www.amsa.org/div/

Association of American Medical Colleges (AAMC). (1998). Teaching and learning of cultural competence in medical school. *Contemporary Issues in Medical Education*, *1*(5), 1–2.

Berger, P. L., & Luckmann, T. (1966). *The social construction of reality*. New York: Doubleday.

Bonecutter, F. J., & Gleeson, J. P. (1997). Broadening our view: Lessons from kinship foster care. *Journal of Multicultural Social Work*, *5*(1–2), 99–119.

Brown, D. E. (1991). *Human universals*. Philadelphia: Temple University Press.

Bureau of Labor Statistics. (2006, Jan.). Annual averages—household data, 2005. Table 11. Employed persons by detailed occupation, sex, race, and Hispanic or Latino. Retrieved January 22, 2007, from ftp://ftp.bls.gov/pub/special.requests/lf/aat11.txt

Butler, R. O., Hood, R. G., & Jordan, W. C. (2005). Optimizing treatment for African Americans and Latinos with HIV/AIDS. *Journal of the National Medical Association*, *97*(8), 1093–1100.

Campinha-Bacote, J. (1994). Cultural competence in psychiatric nursing: A conceptual model. *Nursing Clinics of North America*, *29*(1), 1–8.

Centers for Disease Control and Prevention (CDC). (2006). *HIV/AIDS surveillance report, 2005.* Vol. 17. Atlanta, GA: U.S. Department of Health and Human Services. Retrieved January 22, 2007, from http://www.cdc.gov/hiv/topics/surveillance/resources/reports/2005report/pdf/2005SurveillanceReport.pdf

Cross, T. L., Bazron, B. J., Dennis, K. W., & Isaacs, M. R. (1989). *Towards a culturally competent system of care: A monograph on effective services for minority children who are severely emotionally disturbed*. Washington, DC: CASSP Technical Assistance Center, Georgetown University Child Development Center.

Dana, R. H., Behn, J. D., & Gonwa, T. (1992). A checklist for the examination of cultural competence in social service agencies. *Research on Social Work Practice*, *2*(2), 220–233.

Davis, K. (1997). *Exploring the intersection between cultural competency and managed behavioral health care policy: Implications for state and county mental health agencies*. Alexandria, VA: National Technical Assistance Center for State Mental Health Planning.

Day, J. C. (1996). Population projections of the United States by age, sex, race, and Hispanic origin: 1995 to 2050. (*Current Population Reports*, P25–1130.) Washington, DC: U.S. Bureau of the Census. Retrieved May 22, 2005, from http://www.census.gov/prod/1/pop/p25–1130/p251130.pdf

Diaz, R. M., Ayala, G., & Marín, B. V. (2000). Latino gay men and HIV: Risk behavior as a sign of oppression. *Focus: A Guide to AIDS Research and Counseling*, *15*(7), 1–4.

Diaz, R. (1998). *Latino gay men and HIV: Culture, sexuality and risk behavior*. Boston: Routledge Kegan Paul.

Flores, G. (1997, Nov–Dec). Improving quality through cross-cultural medical practice. *California Family Physician*, 9–17.

Fortier, J. P., Convissor, R., & Pacheco, G. (1999). *Assuring cultural competence in health care: Recommendations for national standards and an outcomes-focused research agenda*. Washington, DC: U.S. Department of Health and Human Services, Resources for Cross Cultural Health Care.

Geertz, C. (1973). *The interpretation of cultures*. New York: Basic Books.

Gómez, C. A., & Marín, B. V. (1996). Gender, culture, and power: Barriers to HIV prevention strategies. *Journal of Sex Research*, *33*(4), 355–362.

Grant, D., & Haynes, D. (1995). A developmental framework for cultural competence training with children. *Social Work in Education*, *17*(3), 171–182.

Grieco, E. M. (2001, Aug). The white population: 2000. *Census 2000 Brief*. January 16, 2006, from http://www.census.gov/prod/2001pubs/c2kbr01-4.pdf

Health Resources and Services Administration (HRSA), U.S. Department of Health and Human Services. (2001). *Cultural competence works: Using cultural competence to improve the quality of health care for diverse populations and add value to managed care arrangements*. Merrifield, VA: HRSA. Retrieved May 27, 2007, from http://minority-health.pitt.edu/archive/00000278/01/cultural-competence_works-(assessment_tool).pdf

Hoban, M. T., & Ward, M. S. (2003). Building culturally competent college health programs. *Journal of American College Health*, *52*(3), 137–141.

Hofstede, G. H. (2001). *Culture's consequences: Comparing values, behaviors, institutions, and organizations across nations* (2nd ed.). Thousand Oaks, CA: Sage Publications.

Joint United Nations Programme on HIV/AIDS (UNAIDS) & the World Health Organization (WHO). (2006). *AIDS epidemic update: Special report on HIV/AIDS: December 2006*. Geneva, Switzerland: UNAIDS. Retrieved May 27, 2007, from http://data.unaids.org/pub/EpiReport/2006/2006_EpiUpdate_en.pdf

Kelly, J. A., & Kalichman, S. C. (2002). Behavioral research in HIV/AIDS primary and secondary prevention: Recent advances and future directions. *Journal of Consulting and Clinical Psychology*, *70*(3), 626–639.

King, M. A., Sims, A., & Osher, D. (2000). *How is cultural competence integrated in education?* Washington, DC: American Institutes for Research.

Like, R. C., Steiner, R. P., & Rubel, A. J. (1996). STFM core curriculum guidelines: Recommended core curriculum guidelines on culturally sensitive and competent health care. *Family Medicine*, *28*(4), 291–297.

Lipson, J. G., & Dibble, S. L. (Eds.). (2005). *Culture & clinical care*. San Francisco: UCSF Nursing Press.

Lum, D. (2003). *Culturally competent practice: A framework for understanding diverse groups and justice issues*. Pacific Grove, CA: Brooks/Cole.

Marín, B. V. (2003). HIV prevention in the Hispanic community: Sex, culture, and empowerment. *Journal of Transcultural Nursing*, *14*(3), 186–192.

Marín, B. V., Gómez, C. A., & Hearst, N. (1993). Multiple heterosexual partners and condom use among Hispanics and non-Hispanic Whites. *Family Planning Perspectives*, *25*(4), 170–174.

Markus, H. R., & Kitayama, S. (1991). Culture and the self: Implications for cognition, emotion, and motivation. *Psychological Review*, *98*(2), 224–253.

Marsiglia, F. F., & Navarro, R. (1999). Acculturation status and HIV/AIDS knowledge and perception of risk among a group of Mexican American middle school students. *Journal of HIV/AIDS Prevention and Education for Adolescents and Children*, *3*(3), 43–61.

McManus, M. C. (1988). Services to minority populations: What does it mean to be a culturally competent professional? *Focal Point*, *2*(4), 1–9.

Office of Minority Health (OMH), U.S. Department of Health and Human Services. (2001). *National standards for culturally and linguistically appropriate services in health care: Final report*. Washington, DC: OMH. Retrieved January 16, 2006, from http://www.omhrc.gov/assets/pdf/checked/finalreport.pdf

Raj, A., Amaro, H., & Reed, E. (2001). Culturally tailoring HIV/AIDS prevention programs: Why, when, and how. In S. S. Kazarian & D. R. Evans (Eds.), *Handbook of cultural health psychology* (pp. 195–239). San Diego, CA: Academic Press.

Santos, G., Puga, A. M., & Medina, C. (2004). HAART, adherence, and cultural issues in the US Latino community. *The AIDS Reader*, *14*(10 Suppl), S26–S29.

Scheer, J. (1994). Culture and disability: An anthropological point of view. In E. J. Trickett, R. J. Watts, & D. Birman (Eds.), *Human diversity: Perspectives on people in context* (pp. 244–260). San Francisco: Jossey-Bass.

Schilder, A. J., Kennedy, C., Goldstone, I. L., Ogden, R. D., Hogg, R. S., & O'Shaughnessy, M. V. (2001). "Being dealt with as a whole person." Care-seeking and adherence: The benefits of culturally competent care. *Social Science and Medicine*, *52*(11), 1643–1659.

Scott, K. D., Gilliam, A., & Braxton, K. (2005). Culturally competent HIV prevention strategies for women of color in the United States. *Health Care for Women International*, *26*(1), 17–45.

Smedley, B. D., Adrienne, Y. S., & Nelson, A. R. (Eds.). (2002). *Unequal treatment: Confronting racial and ethnic disparities in healthcare*. Washington, DC: National Academies Press.

Sowers-Hoag, K. M., & Sandau-Beckler, P. (1996). Educating for cultural competence in the generalist curriculum. *Journal of Multicultural Social Work*, *4*(3), 37–56.

Stevenson, H. C., & White, J. J. (1994). AIDS prevention struggles in ethnocultural neighborhoods: Why research partnerships with community based organizations can't wait. *AIDS Education and Prevention*, *6*(2), 126–139.

Stone, V., Mauch, M., & Steger, K. A. (1998). Provider attitudes regarding participation of women and person of color in AIDS clinical trials. *Journal of Acquired Immune Deficiency Syndromes and Human Retrovirology*, *19*(3), 245–253.

Sue, S. (1998). In search of cultural competence in psychotherapy and counseling. *American Psychologist*, *53*(4), 440–448.

Sue, S., & Zane, N. (1987). The role of culture and cultural techniques in psychotherapy: A critique and reformulation. *American Psychologist*, *42*(1), 37–45.

Suh, E. E. (2004). The model of cultural competence through an evolutionary concept analysis. *Journal of Transcultural Nursing*, *15*(2), 93–102.

Valleroy, L. A., MacKellar, D. A., Karon, J. M., Janssen, R. S., & Hayman, C. R. (1998). HIV infection in disadvantaged out-of-school youth: Prevalence for US Job Corps entrants, 1990 through 1996. *Journal of Acquired Immune Deficiency Syndromes and Human Retrovirology*, *19*(1), 67–73.

Vinh-Thomas, P., Bunch, M. M., & Card, J. J. (2003). A research-based tool for identifying and strengthening culturally competent and evaluation-ready HIV/AIDS prevention programs. *AIDS Education and Prevention, 15*(6), 481–498.

Wilson, B. D. M., & Miller, R. L. (2003). Examining strategies for culturally grounded HIV prevention: A review. *AIDS Education and Prevention, 15*(2), 184–202.

Zenilman, J. M., Shahmanesh, M., & Winter, A. J. (2001). Ethnicity and STIs: More than black and white. *Sexually Transmitted Infections, 77*(1), 2–3.

## Tools and Other Resources for Assessing Cultural Competence at the Individual (i.e., Staff Member) Level

National Center for Cultural Competence. Self-assessment checklist for personnel providing primary health care services. Retrieved May 22, 2005, from http://gucchd.georgetown.edu/nccc/nccc11.html

Management Science for Health. (n.d.). Quality & culture quiz. Retrieved May 23, 2005, from http://erc.msh.org/quiz.cfm?action=question&qt=all&module=provider

Wisconsin's HIV Prevention Community Planning Council. (1999). Multicultural competency self-assessment for prevention service providers. Retrieved May 22, 2005, from http://www.wihivpts.wisc.edu/libraryDownload.asp?docid=122

## Tools and Other Resources for Assessing Cultural Competence at the Agency Level

Andrulis, D., Delbanco, T., Avakian, L., & Shaw-Taylor, Y. (n.d.). Conducting a cultural competence self-assessment. Retrieved May 19, 2005, from http://erc.msh.org/provider/andrulis.pdf

Child Welfare League of America. (1993). Cultural competence self-assessment instrument. Washington, DC: Child Welfare League of America.

Dana, R. H., Behn, J. D., & Gonwa, T. (1992). A checklist for the examination of cultural competence in social service agencies. *Research on Social Work Practice, 2*(2), 220–233.

HIV Prevention Planning Council. (1999). Assessing cultural competency among providers. *San Francisco HIV prevention plan, 1997 and 1998,* Condensed version, pp. 70–78. Retrieved May 27, 2005, from http://www.dph.sf.ca.us/HIVPrevPlan/page2.htm

National Center for Cultural Competence. (2002; Winter). A guide to planning and implementing organizational self-assessment. Retrieved May 22, 2005, from http://gucchd.georgetown.edu/nccc/documents/ncccorgselfassess.pdf

Office of Minority Health (OMH), U.S. Department of Health and Human Services. (2001). *National standards for culturally and linguistically appropriate services in health care: Final report.* Washington, DC: OMH. Retrieved January 16, 2006, from http://www.omhrc.gov/assets/pdf/checked/finalreport.pdf

Work Group on Health Promotion and Community Development at the University of Kansas. Community Tool Box. Retrieved May 22, 2005, from http://ctb.ku.edu/index.jsp

# Culturally Competent Program Planning

## OVERVIEW

*Culturally competent program planning* involves taking a "look inward" at staff and agency norms, values, and assumptions; considering the social, economic, and cultural factors that influence the target population's HIV risk-related behavior and access to prevention services; and striving to create services that are appropriate for and accepted by the target community. A number of key activities are essential to this process. These activities are summarized first and then discussed in greater detail in the remainder of this section.

### Assessing Needs and Assets

HIV-related *needs and assets assessment* is the process of collecting and assessing data that describe the nature and magnitude of a target community's HIV-related needs and resources. The information that is collected should describe: the extent, magnitude, and scope of the HIV-related problem in the target community; current efforts to address the problem; gaps in existing services; local residents' perceptions of the problem's causes and potential solutions; and current science-based knowledge about "what works" to prevent the problem. Needs and assets assessment should include a focus on cultural issues that influence HIV risk behaviors and affect access to and use of HIV prevention-related services.

### Identifying and Involving Community Leaders

Involving *community leaders* in program planning can help make your prevention efforts more culturally competent and thereby increase community support for—and participation in—the program. Community leaders can contribute to program planning by: participating in focus groups or community meetings that provide input on the target population's needs and assets; serving as members of program planning committees; and serving as advocates who champion the program with policy makers or community groups.

## Defining the Problem

Once you have conducted needs and assets assessment with community leader assistance, it is helpful to summarize the findings in a succinct *problem statement* that can serve as a basis for subsequent HIV prevention program planning efforts. The statement should include: your vision with respect to the problem's origins and solution; a description of the affected population; evidence for the scope of the problem; a description of the problem's probable causes and ideas about how to address them; and a few indicators of a successful intervention effort. It should also reflect culturally-specific HIV prevention needs of the target population and community.

## Applying Formal Behavioral and Social Theories

*Formal behavioral and social theories* comprise principles and models about learning and behavior that have proven useful in explaining behavior or in designing effective interventions in health or social areas. Formal theories can be used individually or in combination to provide a program development framework. Examples of theories that have been shown to underlie effective HIV prevention interventions include the Harm Reduction Model, Health Belief Model, Stages of Change Model, Theory of Reasoned Action, Social Learning Theory/Social Cognitive Theory, and Diffusion of Innovations Theory.

## Identifying Goals and Objectives

Before starting to plan program content, it is important to decide on program *goals* and *objectives*—what you want to change in program clients over the long term and short term, respectively. Long-term goals generally focus on behavioral and health status changes, whereas short-term objectives usually focus on the changes in knowledge, attitudes, skills, and intentions that you think will lead to the desired behavioral and health status changes. Goals and objectives should reflect the community needs in your problem statement and should be specific, realistic, and measurable. Program staff and members of the target population and community should provide input into goal and objective development to help ensure their cultural appropriateness.

## Planning Program Components

*Program components* are the HIV prevention activities or services that are designed to achieve your goals and objectives. Key dimensions of program components include the prevention approach, content, delivery methods, duration and frequency, delivery setting, and staffing. Program components should be linked to program objectives and goals. When program staff and community members provide input into program component development, they can help ensure that components reflect your target group's cultural needs.

## Developing and Using Program Models

A *program model* (or *logic model*) is a visual representation of your program's goals and objectives and the program components that you will employ to achieve them. Your model should reflect your target population's needs and assets, your agency's philosophy and resources, and research-based approaches to HIV prevention. Program modeling can help you develop or adapt a program to address local needs; achieve consensus on and commitment to program design among diverse stakeholders; identify weaknesses in program design; allocate resources across program components; identify what program "success" would look like from process and outcome perspectives; and communicate with others about your program.

## Replicating Existing Programs Versus Developing New Programs

*Replication* is the process of moving an intervention to a new site in a way that maintains faithfulness to the underlying theory, overarching goals, and principal components but also permits adaptation to the new context. Replicating a program that has shown positive effects at another site can save staff from having to "reinvent the wheel." A well-chosen, carefully planned program that is implemented with fidelity to its original developer's intent and design has a much greater likelihood of achieving positive outcomes. However, needs and resources differ across communities and agencies. It is therefore important to consider carefully whether replicating a program, developing a new program, or developing a hybrid program would be best for the new context.

## Adapting Programs

Many potential sources of mismatch may make an existing program's approach, content, delivery methods, or required staffing inappropriate for your target population, agency, or community context. For example, the literacy level of your clients may be lower than the level of clients in the original program. *Adaptation* is a process of altering a program to reduce mismatches between that program and the new implementation context. When adapting a program that has shown positive effects in another site, it is important to retain fidelity to the *core program*. Using a program model to make systematic adaptations can facilitate this process. Involving program staff and target population representatives in the adaptation effort is essential to planning a program that appropriately addresses local HIV-related needs.

## Recruiting and Training Staff

The skill and dedication of program staff are vital to program success. Agency managers, current staff, and members of the program's target population should all provide input on new program position descriptions and, as appropriate, participate in reviewing candidates. Candidates should believe in the program's goals and methods and be able to work effectively with existing program staff and the program's target population. All program staff should be trained in program content and delivery methods, how to complete evaluation-related documentation, and issues pertaining to cultural competence, such as how to be more aware of their own and others' cultural values, and techniques for communicating more effectively with clients of different backgrounds.

## ASSESSING NEEDS AND ASSETS

## What Is Needs and Assets Assessment?

*Needs and assets assessment* can be defined as the process of collecting and assessing data that describe the nature and magnitude of a community's needs in relation to an issue, as well as its relevant resources or assets (e.g., financial, organizational, intellectual, institutional, and human) (Card et al., 2001). The information that is collected should address:

1. The extent, magnitude, and scope of the problem in the community.
2. Current efforts and resources to address the problem.
3. Gaps in existing services.
4. Local residents' perceptions of the problem, its causes, and its potential solutions.
5. Current science-based knowledge about "what works" to prevent the problem.

## How Assessing Needs and Assets Can Further Cultural Competence

In the context of HIV prevention, needs and assets assessment should include a focus on cultural issues that influence HIV risk behaviors and affect access to and use of HIV prevention-related services. Examples of these issues include: beliefs and values about sexual behavior, drug-related behavior, health, illness, and health services; gender norms; family structure and power dynamics; and languages spoken and literacy levels. Understanding these factors will help you to identify program goals, objectives, and strategies that build on community assets, address target population needs, and reduce barriers to active program participation.

## Other Benefits of Needs and Assets Assessment

Needs and assets assessment can benefit program planning efforts in other ways, as well. Examples of these benefits include: generating interest among community members in program efforts; providing pre-program data that can be used later to evaluate program effects; and justifying resource requests to agency leadership and external funders.

## Needs and Assets Assessment Methods

An effective needs and assets assessment requires some careful planning. Some key steps in this process are included here, along with the accompanying tool(s) that can help.

1. Decide whom to involve
   Tool 2–1: Who Can Help With Community Needs and Assets Assessment?
2. Identify questions to be addressed
   Tool 2–2: Sample Questions for a Needs and Assets Assessment
   Tool 2–3: What Questions Do We Want Our Needs and Assets Assessment to Answer?
3. Determine what data to collect and how to analyze it
   Tool 2–4: Sources of Needs and Assets Data
   Tool 2–5: Needs and Assets Data Collection and Analysis Planning Matrix
4. Decide whom to disseminate findings to, and how
   Tool 2–6: Matrix for Disseminating Needs and Assets Assessment Findings

It is important to be aware that in many cases, relevant data are already available through government censuses and surveys, public health department reports, research articles in reputable journals, and needs assessment and evaluation reports prepared by other agencies. If you need to collect new data, then surveys, interviews, focus groups, and community forum events may be useful methods to employ.

*Surveys* enable you to obtain information about the opinions, attitudes, and self-reported behaviors of many individuals on a given topic, using a standard set of questions. These questions may be posed on paper, on a computer screen, or orally. *Interviews* may be conducted in-person or by phone, usually at a location that is convenient to the interviewee (such as an office or home). They typically reach fewer people than surveys, but may yield more in-depth information. In *semistructured interviews,* the interviewer uses a list of broad questions to guide the interview but also poses follow-up questions (or *prompts*) that encourage more specific and detailed responses. *Focus groups* are small discussion groups (typically composed of 5–10 people) led by a trained facilitator. They can be used to provide insight into a target population's perceptions and beliefs, find out what language is commonly used in the community to talk about an issue, and test new concepts. They can

The needs and assets assessment data collection methods you choose should be tailored to:
- The questions being addressed.
- Local community characteristics (e.g., literacy levels, preferred communication channels).
- Resources available for the assessment.

For example, suppose that your question is, "What populations in our community are not being served by existing HIV prevention programming?" If you have the resources available, you may want to conduct a survey of local service agencies to determine what HIV prevention services they offer for different populations. With more limited resources, you can still conduct research via the Internet or call several larger service agencies to find out what local services they offer or are aware of.

**Figure 2-1  Tips: Selecting needs and assets assessment data collection methods.**

also be used to test questions in draft evaluation surveys or interview protocols (see also Table 4–1 in Section 4). *Community forums* are community meetings convened by government agencies, private nonprofit organizations, or coalitions to gather community members' opinions about key issues or strategies. Some forums rely on more formal presentation of initial needs and assets assessment information by a speaker or panel, followed by an opportunity for questions and answers and public discussion. Other forums allow anyone to speak for up to a specified period of time. Community forum events typically have designated note-takers. Sometimes forum participants are also encouraged to provide written feedback on special comment cards.

Figure 2–1 provides some additional needs and assets assessment tips. Several of the methods and benefits of needs and assets assessment are exemplified in Tale 2–1, which describes activities that led to development of an effective HIV prevention video for inner-city Hispanics in New York.

## IDENTIFYING AND INVOLVING COMMUNITY LEADERS

### Who Are Community Leaders?

A *community* is a group of persons with common characteristics or interests. Communities can be defined by location, occupation, cultural affiliation, interest in particular issues or activities, shared experiences, or other common bonds (Florida Dept. of Health, 2004). A *community leader* can be anyone who is identified by members of a group as their representative or as someone they respect, such as policy makers and elected officials, community organizers and activists, neighborhood committee members, religious and spiritual leaders, community elders, or *opinion leaders* (i.e., people who others look up to) among peer groups. It is important to be aware that some opinion leaders may not fit the traditional profile of a community leader, particularly if they are members of very narrow or highly marginalized groups. For example, opinion leaders among sex workers, homeless or street populations, or injection drug users may not be quoted in newspapers or other media, have political power, or have name recognition outside their specific communities. However, the breadth and depth of their influence within their communities may afford them a crucial role in HIV prevention efforts.

### Why Involving Community Leaders in Program Planning Is Important

It is important that the needs and interests of the community be represented in all aspects of HIV prevention programming. Involving community leaders in program planning (and program implementation and evaluation) can help make your prevention efforts more culturally competent. This can, in turn, increase community

## 2-1   Developing Video-Based Patient Education for Inner-City Hispanics

Lydia O'Donnell and her colleagues at the Education Development Center were concerned about the high rates of sexually transmitted infections (STIs), including HIV, among inner-city Hispanics in New York. The team understood that although STI clinics had the potential to reach many patients with prevention messages, they often had limited time and resources. Few clinics had sufficient numbers of bilingual/bicultural staff, and most faced a shortage of materials designed to meet the language and cultural needs of Hispanic clients.

O'Donnell and her team wanted to develop an effective STI/HIV intervention program, designed specifically for Hispanics. They decided to take a video-based approach, and they used needs and assets assessment research to collect information that would help ensure that the intervention would be culturally sensitive and relevant to the target population (O'Donnell et al., 1994).

In carrying out needs and assets assessment, the researchers first identified some key questions that they wanted answered by the people who would hopefully one day use the video—Hispanics living in the South Bronx and Queens, New York, and the clinic staff who served them. These questions included:

- How do cultural values, beliefs and attitudes influence Hispanics' willingness to use condoms in different situations?
- How do gender and culture together influence Hispanics' willingness to use condoms in different situations (for example, the idea that Latinos may feel it isn't macho or manly to use condoms)?
- What levels of knowledge and misinformation about STIs/HIV exist among Hispanics in these communities?

The team used a variety of methods to collect their data, including focus groups, personal interviews, and surveys with clinic patients. They also interviewed STI clinic staff and observed interactions between patients and staff in these settings. They found that, among the population studied, (1) discussions about sex and protection between partners tended to be limited; (2) there was little motivation to change these communication patterns; and (3) knowledge about condoms and some aspects of HIV and other STIs was limited.

Next, the researchers teamed up with clinic staff and video producers to talk about these findings and begin developing a video script. They decided that the script and video format would be modeled after popular *telenovelas*—soap operas—and would include characters and scenarios familiar to the Hispanic community. The video would be produced mainly in Spanish, but English lines would be included so that all key messages would appear in both languages.

Building on what they had learned in their needs and assets assessment research, the program developers decided to have the video show examples of condom use behaviors that did not involve a lot of talking between the characters. They also used culturally familiar family and peer conversations to convey information about STIs and HIV. Some of the videos depicted scenes involving men and women, some only men, and others only women. All scripts were written in ways that illustrated culturally specific beliefs about gender roles.

The video came to life with input from many people. Once the script was developed, it was reviewed by experts in STI prevention and health education, as well as by members of the local community. Actors were hired, and a rehearsal was held at a local Hispanic community center. The audience provided further input to the script. After the video was filmed, it was pilot-tested with English-speaking, Spanish-speaking, and bilingual audiences. The final product, *Porque Sí* (*Just Because*), is 18 minutes long.

Could this video intervention, which was developed in accordance with needs and assets assessment findings, really make a difference? O'Donnell and her research team conducted what is called an *outcome study* of the *Porque Sí* video intervention to try to answer that question (O'Donnell et al., 1995). In the study, STI clinic patients were randomly assigned to one of three groups: (1) patients who received only regular clinic services, (2) patients who viewed the video, and (3) patients who viewed the video and then participated in an interactive session with a facilitator. Compared to the patients who received only regular clinic services, video viewers showed greater knowledge of condoms and STIs, more positive attitudes about condom use, increased condom carrying, greater understanding of STI/HIV risks, and a greater ability to make sexual health decisions in their best interests. Some of these positive outcomes were even greater among those who both watched the video and participated in the interactive group session.

*Porque Sí* (*Just Because*) is now a part of the *Voices/Voces* program, which has demonstrated positive effects on condom use behavior and STI infection rates among African-American and Latino adult clinic clients (O'Donnell et al., 1998). For more information on *Voices/Voces*, including how to obtain program materials and training in the program's implementation see Hamdallah et al. (2006), Harshbarger et al. (2006), and http://www.effectiveinterventions. org/interventions/voices_voces.cfm, a Web page of the Centers for Disease Control and Prevention-sponsored Diffusion of Effective Behavioral Interventions (DEBI) Project.

support for the program, as well as increase program attendance or use of services once the program is implemented.

## Identifying Community Leaders

Community leaders can be identified in a variety of ways, such as through program staff's existing knowledge of the community, needs and assets assessment activities, contacts at other service agencies, focus groups with agency clients, attendance at or participation in community events or activities, and outreach activities (e.g., conducting interviews at local "hang-outs").

It is important to bear in mind that because members of any community have diverse cultural and social affiliations, not everyone in a given community will agree on who the respected leaders are (Butterfoss et al., 1996). For example, in any given "Latino community," there may be persons of different national origins, socioeconomic classes, language backgrounds (e.g., Spanish-only speakers, bilingual individuals, and English-only speakers), and so on. For this reason, it is important to identify leaders within the various subgroups of your target community, in order to ensure that diverse views are represented.

## Community Leaders as Resources for Program Planning

How might you involve community leaders in program planning efforts? Some examples of important roles that community members can play include:

- Participant in a focus group or community forum meeting that provides input on community needs and assets.
- Member of a program planning committee that provides advice or direction on program design.
- Program advocate who champions the program with policy makers or community groups.

To facilitate your identification and involvement of community leaders, you may wish to use Tool 2-7: Matrix for Involving Community Leaders in Program Planning. An example of the benefits of involving community leaders in program planning and evaluation is provided in Tale 2-2, which describes an HIV prevention intervention designed for male patrons of gay bars.

# 2-2 Using Opinion Leaders at Bars to Communicate HIV Prevention Messages to Men Who Have Sex With Men

Can people with well-respected opinions influence the sexual behaviors of other people?

Jeff Kelly of the Medical College of Wisconsin created a program that sheds light on this question. Kelly and his colleagues designed the *Popular Opinion Leaders* (POL) program to reduce unprotected sex among male patrons of gay bars (Kelly et al., 1991; Kelly et al., 1992). The POL program uses *popular opinion leaders* (i.e., bar patrons that other patrons seem to look up to) to deliver safer sex messages. A key aspect of this strategy is to create the impression that safer sex is the norm among people who are respected and admired.

In the original study of the POL program, Kelly and colleagues went to one or two large gay bars in each of three cities—Biloxi, Mississippi; Monroe, Louisiana; and Hattiesburg, Mississippi. In each setting, the researchers trained the bartenders to identify opinion leaders. For example, bartenders were trained to make note of people who came to the bar frequently and were routinely greeted by other patrons. People who were identified by more than one bartender were then:

- Approached by one of the researchers and told they were identified by others as a highly influential bar patron.
- Asked if they would consider using this influence to possibly save others' lives by delivering safer sex messages to peers.
- Asked to invite another influential friend to participate.

Those who agreed to participate in the program completed several training sessions on how to communicate HIV prevention messages to their peers. Training methods included lectures, group discussions, demonstrations of appropriate messages, and role playing exercises. Opinion leaders then signed a contract to have at least 14 sexual risk reduction conversations with peers at the bar. To help stimulate safer sex conversations, opinion leaders wore eye-catching lapel buttons that matched posters hung in the bars.

Did these opinion leaders actually make a difference? The research team conducted a careful evaluation of the POL intervention program to find out. The program was first run in Biloxi, with Monroe and Hattiesburg serving as comparison sites that had not yet received the intervention. The program was then implemented in Monroe (with Hattiesburg still serving as a comparison site), and finally, in Hattiesburg. Patrons in the bars at all three sites were surveyed at regular intervals.

Reviewing the data, researchers learned that the opinions of the leaders did make a difference. In each city after the POL program had been run, unprotected anal intercourse among bar patrons decreased significantly from the sexual activity levels reported before the intervention. In comparison sites, there was little or no change in sexual risk behavior during the same period (Kelly et al., 1992). A larger study of the program, conducted in eight small U.S. cities, also found that the opinion leaders had a significant positive influence on the sexual risk practices of their peers (Kelly et al., 1997).

The POL intervention has since been adapted for use in other settings, including "hustler" bars (i.e., bars frequented by male prostitutes and their male clients) (Miller, 2003; Miller et al., 1998; see also Tale 2–6) and Latino migrant men who have sex with other men (Somerville et al., 2006).

For more information on POL, including how to obtain program materials and training in POL implementation, see http://www.effectiveinterventions.org/interventions/POL.cfm, a Web page of the Centers for Disease Control and Prevention-sponsored Diffusion of Effective Behavioral Interventions (DEBI) Project.

# DEFINING THE PROBLEM

## What Is a Problem Statement?

Once you have conducted a needs and assets assessment of your local community, it is helpful to summarize your findings in a succinct *problem statement.* A problem statement offers an overview of the issues, problems, and needs facing a community, and it suggests ways to address these needs. It can serve as the basis for further program planning tasks.

## Components of a Problem Statement

A problem statement has six main components (Card et al., 2001):

1. **Your vision, point of view, or values with respect to the problem.**
   EXAMPLE: Our vision is that all people in our community will make healthy sexual decisions and avoid infection with HIV.
2. **Definition of the population affected.**
   EXAMPLE: In Newburgh City, young African-American women (ages 19–29) have the highest rate of AIDS diagnosis across all cultural groups.
3. **Evidence for the scope/severity of the problem.**
   EXAMPLE: Over 50% of AIDS cases among Newburgh City residents occur among African-Americans under age 40. One out of 80 African-American females ages 19–29 is HIV+.
4. **Description of the likely causes of the problem and the gaps between needs and available services.**
   EXAMPLE: Due in part to gender-based socialization, young African-American women in our community lack the skills, self-efficacy, and motivation to negotiate safer sex successfully. Few programs offer a safe environment in which to address the factors contributing to HIV infection.
5. **Ideas about how to address the problem, based on current research and community perspectives.**
   EXAMPLE: Young women need opportunities to build skills, self-efficacy and motivation to engage in safer sex practices in ways that are culturally appropriate. Focus groups and the HIV prevention literature suggest that peer educator-led workshops (led by well-trained facilitators) can address this need.
6. **Indicators that would show that the problem has been solved**
   EXAMPLE: We would expect program participants to increase safer sex practices (e.g., condom-protected sex), which will ultimately contribute to lower HIV infection rates in our community.

A brief sample problem statement is provided in Figure 2–2. To develop your own problem statement, you may wish to use Tool 2–8: Problem Statement Development Worksheet.

## Enhancing Cultural Competence in Problem Statement Development

It is important that your problem statement reflect the culturally related HIV prevention needs of your target population and community. To accomplish this, you should involve members of these groups in problem statement development. Specifically, you may wish to hold community forum events, meetings, or focus groups to present the needs and assets assessment findings and get diverse input on problem statement development.

Our vision is that all men and women in our community, Newburgh City, will have the knowledge and skills that they need to make healthy sexual decisions and avoid infection with HIV/AIDS. African Americans in Newburgh City have the highest HIV prevalence rates of all ethnic groups. Among African Americans, young adults (ages 19–29) are at particularly high risk of HIV infection. It is estimated that in Newburgh City, 1 out of 40 males and 1 out of 130 females are HIV+. Over 50% of all HIV infections that occur among Newburgh City residents occur in the African-American community, and 75% of HIV+ persons contracted the virus before age 30 (Newburgh City Public Health Department, 2005).

The high risk of HIV infection in Newburgh City, particularly among African Americans, is a result of a number of factors. African-American teens and young adults lack knowledge about how to protect themselves from HIV. They also lack the skills and motivation to successfully negotiate safer sex with a partner. This is particularly true of young women, who commonly have unprotected sex with a male partner even when they do not want to in order to avoid rejection. Few programs in the community offer teens and young adults a safe, supportive, and culturally sensitive environment in which to acquire the knowledge, skills, and motivation that they need to avoid HIV infection. Yet, there are a number of teens and young adults who make healthy sexual choices and want to share their skills with others for the benefit of the community as a whole.

Teens and young adults need opportunities to build their HIV-related knowledge, communication skills, and motivation to engage in safer sex practices in ways that emphasize ethnic pride, culturally appropriate roles and actions, and strengthening of community. Both focus groups with community members and a review of the HIV prevention literature suggest that peer educator-led workshops for male teens, female teens, male young adults, and female young adults can address this need, as long as workshop facilitators receive proper training in program content and methods. We would expect participants in such a program to show a significant increase in safer sex practices, which will ultimately contribute to lower HIV infection rates in our community.

**Reference**
Newburgh City Public Health Department. (2005). *HIV surveillance in Newburgh City, 1994–2004.* Newburgh City, IL: Epidemiology Unit, Newburgh City Public Health Department.

**Figure 2-2  Sample problem statement.**

## Using Your Problem Statement

A problem statement has many potential uses. It can serve as a starting point for subsequent program planning tasks, such as identification of program goals and objectives, content, and delivery formats. It can also serves as the "background" section for a funding proposal, report to a Board or funder, evaluation report, or presentation to community members.

## APPLYING FORMAL BEHAVIORAL AND SOCIAL THEORIES

### What Are Formal Theories?

Interventions that seek to change health outcomes related to behavior are based on theories. These theories may concern how information, ideas, and practices spread from one person to another or from one society to another; why people behave as they do; how to change behavior; or how to reduce the harmful health consequences of behavior. These theories may have been extensively tested and written about, or they may come from the beliefs and ideas of program developers. *Formal theories* (also sometimes called *behavioral and social science theories*) are made up of assumptions, principles, methods, and models about social relations, learning, and behavior that have been tested and proven useful in explaining behavior and/or in designing effective interventions in health or social areas (Herlocher et al., 1996; Kirby, 2001). Using one or more appropriate formal theories as the basis for an HIV prevention program can help guide program planning and increase the likelihood that the resultant program is effective in achieving the intended outcomes.

Examples of Formal Theories Underlying Effective HIV Prevention Programs*

| Name of Theory | Summary of Theory | Application to HIV Prevention | Example |
|---|---|---|---|
| A. GENERAL MODELS | | | |
| (1) Diffusion of Innovations Theory (Rogers, 1983) | This theory addresses how innovations—ideas, products, and practices that are new or perceived as new—spread within a society or from one society to another. According to the theory, a number of factors determine the extent and speed with which an innovation spreads: (1) Is the innovation better than what it would replace? (2) Is the innovation a good match for the intended audience? (3) Is the innovation easy to use? (4) Can the innovation be tried out before it is adopted? (5) Are the outcomes of the innovation observable or easily measured? Disseminating an innovation through both mass media and interpersonal interactions increases the likelihood that it will be adopted. Opinion leaders (i.e., people whose opinions are respected within a particular community) tend to pay close attention to the media and are often the first to adopt innovations. They then convey the media content and their own interpretations of it to others, thus encouraging wider adoption of the innovation. | HIV prevention programs based on this model commonly train opinion leaders in the targeted community in risk reduction practices, and in outreach techniques for promoting these practices among others. Specifically, the opinion leaders are trained to address the benefits of the risk reduction practice, how to engage in the practice, and how the practice is consistent with other aspects of the target community's lifestyle. | The *Popular Opinion Leader* program (Kelly et al., 1991; Kelly et al., 1992; Kelly et al., 1997; see also Figures 2-3, 2-12, and 3-2) trains opinion leaders among gay male populations to address sexual risk-related norms, attitudes, and behaviors among their peers. The opinion leaders have casual conversations with their peers at gay bars, and in other settings where gay men socialize, about HIV-related misperceptions, the importance of preventing HIV infection, and specific risk reduction strategies. They also recommend that their peers adopt safer sexual behaviors. To help start conversations, the leaders wear buttons with the project logo, which is also on posters hung at the bars. |
| (2) Harm Reduction Model (Brettle, 1991) | This approach does not seek to eliminate or reduce harmful or risky behaviors, but instead focuses on ways to prevent the negative consequences of these behaviors, based on current attitudes and beliefs. | HIV prevention programs that take harm reduction approaches seek to reduce the likelihood that high-risk behaviors such as injection drug use will lead to HIV infection. They do this by providing tools or resources that reduce the likelihood of contact with HIV-infected body fluids during performance of the risky behaviors. | Needle exchange programs make safer injection a viable choice by providing sterile injection drug equipment, such as clean needles, cookers, and filters, to injection drug users. This reduces the likelihood that injection drug use will result in HIV infection (Wodak & Cooney, 2006) |
| (3) Health Belief Model (Rosenstock et al., 1994) | This model was developed in the 1950s to explain why so few people were participating in health-related prevention and treatment programs. The model is based on the assumption that for people to take action to prevent, test for, or treat illness, they have to: (1) believe they are susceptible to the condition; (2) believe the condition has serious consequences; (3) believe taking action would reduce their susceptibility to the condition or its severity; (4) believe the costs of taking action are outweighed by the benefits; (5) be exposed to environmental factors (such as media messages or advice from health providers or peers) that encourage action; and (6) be confident in their ability to perform the action. | HIV prevention programs based on this model focus on increasing perceived vulnerability to HIV, changing beliefs about the severity of AIDS, changing perceptions of the difficulty of taking risk-reducing actions (such as using condoms or clean needles), and building on existing environmental cues, such as knowing someone who has been diagnosed with HIV or AIDS. | *Turning Point* (Siegal et al., 1995) is a one-on-one counseling and small-group HIV risk reduction program for injection drug users and their sexual partners. The program aims to reduce HIV infection by helping participants to recognize the behaviors that put them at risk of HIV infection, the severity of AIDS, and the benefits of risk reduction behaviors. The program also seeks to increase participants' skills and confidence to engage in risk reduction behaviors. |

(*continued*)

## Examples of Formal Theories Underlying Effective HIV Prevention Programs

| Name of Theory | Summary of Theory | Application to HIV Prevention | Example |
|---|---|---|---|
| (4) Social Learning Theory/Social Cognitive Theory (Bandura, 1986) | This theory is based on the notion that individual factors (skills, motivation, and confidence in one's ability to take action) and environmental factors (observational learning, reinforcement by others) and behaviors interact and are interdependent. Confidence in one's ability to take action is considered to be particularly important to engaging in a behavior, as is the observation and interpretation of the behavior as performed by others. | HIV prevention programs based on this theory typically include HIV risk education, sensitization to the threat of HIV/AIDS, enhancement of motivation to reduce HIV risk, and HIV risk reduction skills training. The skills training generally provides an explanation and modeling of the skills, discussion of the model's performance, opportunities for skills practice with corrective feedback, and social support for behavior change. | See Tale 2–3 for several examples. |
| (5) Stages of Change Model (Transtheoretical Model) (Prochaska et al., 1992) | This model describes five stages of behavior change: (1) *Precontemplation,* in which people are unaware of the problem and have no intention to change; (2) *Contemplation,* in which people recognize the need for change and consider change; (3) *Preparation,* in which they intend to change and plan for change; (4) *Action,* in which they initiate change and put new behaviors into practice; and (5) *Maintenance,* in which they sustain new behaviors and address relapses to earlier stages in the change process. Movement from each stage to the next is determined by different cognitive processes; for example, to move from precontemplation to contemplation, awareness of the behavior's consequences must be raised. | HIV prevention programs based on this model seek to match intervention strategies to each client's current place in the process of risk behavior change. For example, for clients in the contemplation stage of condom use, the objective is to increase their motivation to use condoms. In this way, the program can move clients to successive stages and ultimately support maintenance of HIV risk reduction behaviors. | *The Real AIDS Prevention Project (RAPP): A Community-Level HIV Prevention Intervention for Inner-City Women* is based on several formal theories, including the Stages of Change Model (Lauby et al., 2000). One component of the intervention involves one-on-one outreach by peer network volunteers. In these encounters, volunteers determine each woman's stage of change with respect to condom use and motivate her to advance to the next stage, with stage-appropriate messages. The volunteers also distribute brochures with stories of community women in the same stage as the client. |
| (6) Theory of Gender and Power (Connell, 1987) | This theory examines how certain social structures shape the relationships between men and women and the lives that they lead. These social structures (found in the home and in institutions like schools, churches, government agencies, and businesses) include: (1) *The sexual division of labor:* How do men's versus women's work arrangements shape their lives? (2) *The sexual division of power:* What levels of power do men and women have in different areas of life, and what are the consequences of these arrangements? (3) *Social norms and social attachments:* What are a society's expectations and beliefs about women and men's behaviors, including sexual behaviors? How do these expectations and beliefs influence women's and men's lives? | HIV prevention programs based on this model acknowledge that gender-based inequalities can influence sexual communication and behavior, such as negotiating condom use with a partner. Such programs promote gender-specific risk reduction strategies that take existing gender inequalities into consideration. | See Tale 2–3 for several examples. |

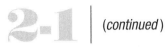 *(continued)*

| Name of Theory | Summary of Theory | Application to HIV Prevention | Example |
|---|---|---|---|
| (7) Theory of Reasoned Action (Fishbein & Ajzen, 1975) and Theory of Planned Behavior (Ajzen, 1988) | According to the *Theory of Reasoned Action*, behavioral intention is the most important determinant of behavior. Behavioral intention is influenced by a person's attitude toward performing the behavior and beliefs about whether others who are important to the person approve or disapprove of the behavior. One limitation of this theory is that it is also based on the premise that behaviors are under the direct control of individuals. The *Theory of Planned Behavior* a variant of the Theory of Reasoned Action, addresses this limitation by adding an additional factor that influences behavioral intentions—*perceived behavioral control*. The assumption is that if people feel that they have a high degree of control over a behavior, they are more likely to intend to perform the behavior. | HIV prevention programs based on these theories focus on the specific personal attitudes, beliefs about social norms, perceived control (in the case of the Theory of Planned Behavior), and behavioral intentions related to each targeted behavior. These attitudes, beliefs, and perceived control will be different for every behavior, such as using a condom with a long-term partner versus with a casual partner. | *Hot, Healthy, and Keeping It Up! (HHKIU)* is a group counseling program for Asian and Pacific Islander gay and bisexual men (Choi et al., 1996). It is based on several formal theories, including the Theory of Reasoned Action. HHKIU seeks to influence attitudes about safer sex behaviors by providing information about HIV/AIDS and safer sex through mini-lectures that focus on the real-life consequences of behavioral choices. In group discussions, participants also gain a clearer idea of what their peers believe about safer sex. Other group activities encourage participants to make decisions and stick to them. |

### B. MODELS SPECIFIC TO HIV PREVENTION

| Name of Theory | Summary of Theory | Application to HIV Prevention | Example |
|---|---|---|---|
| (1) AIDS Risk Reduction Model (AARM) (Catania et al., 1990) | The AARM uses elements of several other models (including the Diffusion of Innovations Theory, Health Belief Model, Social Cognitive Theory, and others) to organize behavior change factors that are specific to HIV risk reduction. It is a stage model comprising three behavioral change steps: (1) recognition of HIV infection risk; (2) commitment to behavior change, which may include changes in attitudes toward the behavior and confidence in one's ability to perform the behavior; and (3) enactment of behavior change, which may include gaining support from others for changing behavior, communicating with others (such as sexual partners) about change, and initiating behavior change. | HIV prevention programs based on this model focus on moving participants through the model's stages by helping participants understand and personalize their risk, changing attitudes toward condom use and/or needle cleaning, building relevant behavioral skills (such as skills to negotiate condom use) and confidence to apply them, and providing social support for behavior change. | *Brother to Brother* is a small-group program for African-American gay and bisexual men (Peterson et al., 1996). The program seeks to increase participants' awareness of their high HIV risk, and build their social support system within the African-American gay/bisexual community. It also teaches safer sex negotiation methods and affords practice through role playing exercises. In addition, participants observe and practice proper condom application. The program also helps participants identify when they are most vulnerable to having unsafe sex and avoid these situations. |
| Information-Motivation-Behavioral Skills (IMB) Model (Fisher & Fisher, 1992) | This HIV-specific model is based on the assumption that *information* about risk reduction and *motivation* to reduce risk influence each other, and are both necessary to change HIV risk behaviors. The model also states that information and motivation are necessary for the development of risk reduction *skills*, and that these skills also contribute to behavior change. | HIV prevention programs based on this model seek to build the knowledge, motivation, and skills needed to change HIV risk behaviors, such as unprotected sex. | *AIDS Risk Reduction for College Students* (Fisher et al., 1996) seeks to reduce students' risk of HIV and STI infection. The program provides information on transmission routes and risk factors and dispels common myths though a slide show and |

*(continued)*

| Name of Theory | Summary of Theory | Application to HIV Prevention | Example |
|---|---|---|---|
| Information- Motivation- Behavioral Skills (IMB) Model (Fisher & Fisher, 1992) | | | follow-up presentation. To motivate risk reduction behaviors, the program uses a video of interviews with HIV-positive persons who are similar to the students in age, appearance, and sexual history. In addition, small-group discussions led by peer educators focus on positively influencing attitudes and perceived social norms around safer sex. Large group discussions promote support for safer behaviors. The final component teaches safer sex skills, including safer sex communication and condom application, through use of a video, discussion, role play, and penis model. The program ends with a behavioral homework assignment. |

\* The theory summaries in Table 2–1 are based on Herlocher et al., 1996; Kalichman, 1998; National Cancer Institute, 2005; and Wingood & DiClemente, 2000.

## Formal Theories Commonly Used in Effective HIV Prevention Programming

Many effective HIV prevention interventions are based on one or more of the theories and models described in Table 2–1. Additional information on these and other theories is also available from the references at the end of this section.

## Common Factors Addressed by Formal Theories

Theories that guide effective HIV prevention interventions collectively address eight factors that influence behavior (Fishbein et al., 2001):

1. **Intention** to perform the behavior (e.g., intention to use a condom with every sexual partner).
2. Presence of **environmental factors** that constrain the behavior (e.g., access to sterile needles for injecting drugs).
3. **Skills** needed to perform the behavior (e.g., ability to successfully negotiate condom use with a partner).
4. **Attitude** toward performing the behavior (e.g., personal feelings about unprotected anal sex).
5. Perception of **social pressure** to perform the behavior (e.g., beliefs about whether peers would approve of condom use).

## 2-3   Using Formal Theories to Develop Effective HIV Prevention Programs for African-American Women

Effective health prevention and promotion programs usually draw on theories that describe the forces and factors influencing human behavior. This is the case for three effective HIV prevention interventions targeting African-American women:

- *SiSTA*—designed for African-American women ages 18–29 (DiClemente & Wingood, 1995).
- *SiHLE*—designed for African-American young women ages 14–18 (DiClemente et al., 2004).
- *WiLLOW*—designed for HIV-positive women ages 18–50 and originally tested with a largely African-American sample (Wingood et al., 2004).

The *SiSTA*, *SiHLE*, and *WiLLOW* programs were designed by Ralph DiClemente, Gina Wingood, and their colleagues at Emory University. The programs—which have been shown to reduce sexual risk behaviors—were developed with insights from two social-behavioral theories:

1. *Social Cognitive Theory* (Bandura, 1994) argues that behavior influences and is influenced by a combination of *individual (or personal) factors* and *environmental factors*. Individual factors include our knowledge, skills, self-confidence and expectations. Environmental factors include the ways we learn by observing others' actions, and seeing the results of those actions. The *SiSTA*, *SiHLE*, and *WiLLOW* programs consider the influence of individual and environmental factors on women's sexual behaviors/choices by:
   □ Offering learning activities that help participants build positive attitudes and skills concerning safer sex behaviors.
   □ Modeling safer sex strategies that participants can first observe and then practice (e.g., proper application of condoms, and culturally appropriate, assertive communication skills that can be used by women when negotiating safer sex).

2. *The Theory of Gender and Power* (Connell, 1987) examines how certain social structures shape the relationships between men and women. These social structures (found in social settings like the home, and in social organizations and institutions such as a church, government, or business) include:
   □ *The sexual division of labor* (e.g., how does work come to be defined as men's work or women's work? How do these work arrangements shape men's and women's lives?)
   □ *The sexual division of power* (e.g., what levels of power do men and women have in different areas of life, and why? What are the consequences of this arrangement?)
   □ *Social norms and social attachments* (e.g., what are a society's expectations and beliefs about women and men's behaviors? Their sexuality? How are women's and men's sexuality related to other aspects of their life, such as family and work?)

Connell's theory helps shed light on the ways that gender-based inequalities can affect our personal relationships and behaviors (e.g., feeling less able to negotiate safer sex practices with our partners). These factors can affect our health, and increase the likelihood of HIV infection (Wingood & DiClemente, 2000).

Building on these theories, the *SiSTA*, *SiHLE*, and *WiLLOW* programs recognize that it can be difficult for women to negotiate consistent condom use if they are in a relationship in which they don't feel equal to their male partner. The programs address challenges that women may face in taking control of their sexual and reproductive health, and offer activities designed to help them address these challenges. Sample activities include:

- Discussing the joys and challenges of being an African-American woman and the accomplishments of African-American women in society to promote gender pride.

■ Building skills to communicate effectively with a male partner about safer sex.

■ Discussing the impact of gender-based violence and abuse on HIV risk and providing follow-up referrals to counseling and shelters to women in unhealthy relationships.

■ Assisting women in fostering and maintaining healthy social support from others in their social networks.

Replication kits for *SiSTA* and *WiLLOW* are available through Sociometrics' HIV/AIDS Prevention Program Archive (HAPPA)—see http://www.

socio.com/pasha/haprogms.htm. A replication kit for *SiHLE* is available through Sociometrics' Program Archive on Sexuality, Health and Adolescence (PASHA)—see http://www.socio.com/srch/summary/pasha/passt23.htm.

For information about training in *SiSTA*, *SiHLE*, and *WiLLOW*, see Wingood and DiClemente (2006) and http://www.effectiveinterventions.org/interventions/sista.cfm, a Web page of the Centers for Disease Control and Prevention-sponsored Diffusion of Effective Behavioral Interventions (DEBI) Project.

6. Perception of the behavior's consistency or inconsistency with **self-image** (e.g., whether one sees oneself as the kind of person who would plan for sex by carrying condoms).

7. **Emotional reaction** to performing the behavior (e.g., whether one feels "empowered" or "disgusted" by the idea of using a dental dam or condom for oral sex).

8. **Self-efficacy**, or the belief in one's ability to perform the behavior in different circumstances (e.g., confidence in one's ability to say "no" to unprotected sex with a primary partner).

## Using Formal Theories in Culturally Competent Ways

Once you have defined the problem to address, consider which theory or theories might be most appropriate for your context. Then use these as guides as you take the next steps in program planning: identifying specific program goals and objectives, developing or adapting program components, and developing your program model. An example of how two formal theories were applied to development of a suite of culturally competent HIV prevention programs for African-American women is provided in Tale 2–3.

## IDENTIFYING GOALS AND OBJECTIVES

## What Are Goals and Objectives?

In program planning, it is tempting to focus first on the activities or services you would like to offer to your clients, and only later to think about your *long-term goals* and *short-term objectives*—what you hope your program will change or achieve among your target population (Card et al., 2001). However, if you define your goals and objectives first, you can then develop activities and services that are focused on achieving them. This will streamline resource use and maximize the likelihood of positive program outcomes.

A comparison of long-term goals and short-term objectives is provided in Table 2–2.

It is often helpful for program planners to also define *mid-term objectives,* which are intermediate changes that you would like to achieve in your target population. Mid-term objectives are expected to result from the short-term objectives and lead

| Comparison of Short-Term Objectives and Long-Term Goals

| Short-term objectives should | Long-term goals should |
|---|---|
| ■ Reflect short-term changes in your target population that will likely lead to program goals. | ■ Reflect the ultimate aims of the program with respect to the target population. |
| ■ Focus on HIV-related knowledge, skills, attitudes, intentions, and (sometimes) behaviors. | ■ Focus on HIV-related behaviors and/or health impacts (e.g., STI infection, HIV serostatus). |
| ■ Be numerous. | ■ Be few in number (i.e., one to three) |
| ■ Be measurable immediately upon participants' completion of a program or up to a few months later. | ■ Be measurable only over long follow-up periods (typically a year or more after program completion). |
| ■ EXAMPLE: To increase condom use negotiation skills. | ■ EXAMPLE: To decrease the incidence of HIV infection by 20% in New City within 4 years. |

to the long-term goals. As is shown in Figure 2–3, if you choose to define three sets of desired outcomes for your program (short-, mid-, and long-term), instead of only two (short- and long-term), the long-term goals should focus on health outcomes, such as infection with HIV or other sexually transmitted infections (STIs). The mid-term objectives generally focus on the key HIV risk or protective behaviors that the program seeks to change, such as use of condoms, frequency of sex, number of sexual partners, use of injection drugs, and the sharing or cleaning of injection drug use equipment. These are the behaviors that are most closely tied to HIV infection risk. The short-term objectives focus on factors that influence these key mid-term behaviors, such as knowledge, attitudes, beliefs, skills, and intentions. Behaviors that influence the mid-term behaviors, such as communicating with sexual partners about safer sex, carrying condoms, and acquiring clean needles, may also be the focus of short-term objectives.

It is important to bear in mind that whether a desired behavioral outcome is short-term, mid-term, or long-term depends on the particular target population that you are working with. For example, if you are planning an HIV prevention program for adults who are sexually active, then the desired outcome of increasing condom use can reasonably be measured in the short term or mid-term. However, if you planning an HIV prevention program for young teens who are, on the whole, not yet sexually active, then the desired outcome of increasing condom use can reasonably be measured only in the long term, once the youth have become sexually active.

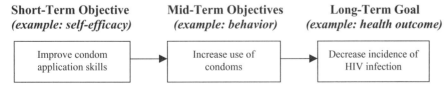

**Short-Term Objective**  *(example: self-efficacy)*    **Mid-Term Objectives**  *(example: behavior)*    **Long-Term Goal**  *(example: health outcome)*

Improve condom application skills → Increase use of condoms → Decrease incidence of HIV infection

**Figure 2-3 Examples of short- and mid-term objectives and a corresponding long-term goal.**

**Examples of Specific, Realistic, and Measurable Objectives/Goals**

| Specific | Realistic | Measurable |
|---|---|---|
| **Not specific:** Increase communication skills | **Not likely realistic:** By three months after the end of the program, 100% of clients will use condoms every time they have sex | **Less measurable:** HIV will be less of a problem in the community |
| **More specific:** Increase ability to successfully negotiate condom use with a partner | **May be more realistic:** By three months after the end of the program, consistent use of condoms will increase by at least 30% among clients | **More measurable:** The diagnosis rate for new HIV infections will decrease by 20% within 4 years |

It is also important to ensure that program goals and objectives are *SMART*—that is, maximally *s*pecific, *m*easurable, *a*ttainable, *r*ealistic, and *t*imely. Goals and objectives that are *specific* are focused and well-defined. When they are *measurable*, it is possible to determine whether they have been achieved. It is also important for goals and objectives to be *attainable* and *realistic*, given the available resources (such as funding, staffing, facilities, and time available to work with the target population). To be considered *timely*, goals and objectives should have an appropriate, well-specified time frame for their attainment. Having SMART goals and objectives increases the likelihood that program success can be achieved and documented.

## Steps for Identifying Culturally Competent Goals and Objectives

The following steps can help ensure that your goals and objectives reflect the HIV-related needs and concerns of your target population.

1. Call a brainstorming meeting with staff and members of your target population or community. Have your problem statement available for reference.
2. Brainstorm and prioritize potential goals and objectives, based on the group's input and research about your population or similar groups. The goals and objectives you identify should address the target population's needs and assets, including their developmental level and HIV risk level. They should also be acceptable to your agency and community.
3. If your program seeks to address multiple populations (e.g., both youth and their parents), set separate goals and objectives for each population.
4. Link objectives to goals in a logical manner. An objective of "increasing the ability to negotiate condom use," for example, links logically to the goal of "increasing condom use."
5. Ensure alignment of objectives and goals with your problem statement and any formal theories that underlie your intervention.
6. Review goals and objectives to ensure that they are SMART—specific, measurable, attainable, realistic, and timely—as this will facilitate your evaluation planning process later on. Examples of less and more specific, realistic, and measurable goals and objectives are provided in Table 2–3.

Dimensions of Program Components

| Feature | Definition | Examples | Cultural factors to consider |
|---|---|---|---|
| Approach | The strategy to be employed | ■ HIV education<br>■ HIV counseling and testing<br>■ Needle exchange<br>■ Outreach | Certain approaches may be more effective than others with particular cultural groups; for example, outreach may be the best way to reach a specific homeless/street population or commercial sex worker population |
| Content | Topics to be covered | ■ How to negotiate safer sex<br>■ How to clean a needle<br>■ Where to get an HIV test | Some cultural groups may be more or less comfortable than others with particular sexual or drug use topics; the way these topics are presented, and the images, language, and examples used, should reflect clients' norms and values |
| Delivery methods | The format, technique, or medium used to deliver the service | ■ One-on-one counseling<br>■ Role-play<br>■ Video | Some cultural groups may be more comfortable than others with group versus one-on-one delivery formats, and with activities such as group discussions or role plays; in addition, for group-based programs, single-sex groups may be crucial for enabling clients of some cultural backgrounds to participate fully |
| Duration & frequency | The length of time and frequency with which services are offered | ■ Workshop series that includes three 1-hour sessions taught once a week for 3 weeks | Cultural norms and values can influence how much time—and what time of day or day of the week—men, women, or youth may be available to participate in programs |
| Setting | The type of location in which the service will be delivered | ■ School classroom<br>■ Clinic<br>■ Community-based organization | Cultural groups may vary with respect to their physical access to particular types of program facilities, as well as with respect to their comfort in using those facilities; for some groups, a less formal setting, such as a community center or private home, may facilitate program participation |
| Staffing | The number, roles, time commitment, and credentials of program staff | ■ 2 Certified Health Education Specialists, each 50% time, to provide HIV education<br>■ 1 phlebotomist to draw blood for HIV testing, 10% time | The match between the cultural and language background of staff and that of clients should always be taken into consideration; in addition, some cultural groups may be more open to receiving information from certain types of people (e.g., men vs. women; older vs. younger people; professional providers or lay workers) |

To develop your goals and objectives, you may wish to use Tool 2–9: Goals and Objectives Planning Worksheet.

# PLANNING PROGRAM COMPONENTS

## What Are Program Components?

*Program components* are the HIV prevention activities or services that you will use or offer to achieve your goals and objectives (Card et al., 2001). Program components can be defined along a number of dimensions, such as those shown in Table 2–4.

Effective behavioral prevention programs include content, delivery methods, and materials that provide opportunities for building *skills* that are appropriate to HIV prevention, such as condom-related communication and negotiation skills (CDC, 2001). Modeling desirable skills and actively engaging participants in role-playing activities are common skills-building approaches. It is important that such activities reflect common sexual or drug use situations that program clients face, such as being pressured for unprotected sex or being offered a dirty needle.

**Figure 2-4  Tip: Effective program components.**

## Steps in Planning Culturally Competent Program Components

The following steps can help ensure that your program components are appropriate for and appealing to your target population.

1. Call a brainstorming meeting involving both staff and members of the target population or community. Have your problem statement and list of goals and objectives available for reference.
2. Brainstorm and prioritize potential program components. This should include discussion of the program component dimensions in Table 2–4. If your intervention will be serving more than one target population (e.g., youth and their parents), be sure to specify which target population will be served by each component.
3. Plan activities and services that reflect:
   □ Target population and community needs, assets, beliefs, and values, such as HIV risk level, developmental level, literacy skills, gender roles and norms, and communication norms.
   □ Agency values and available resources (e.g., mission, staffing, funding, time that can be spent with the target population).
   □ The latest scientific research on effective prevention programming (for example, see the tip in Figure 2–4), including programming for populations that are culturally similar to yours.
4. Link the program components that you define to the program's short-term objectives.

To define your program components, you may wish to use Tool 2–10: Program Components Planning Worksheet.

## Addressing Barriers to Participation

When planning program components, it is also important to consider potential barriers that might prevent clients from attending the program. *Logistical barriers* include inaccessible times or locations, fees that clients cannot afford, or lack of staff who speak clients' languages. *Perceived barriers* include the feeling or belief that the program is not relevant or right for them (Brindis & Davis, 1998). Examples of perceived barriers include discomfort with program staff who are from different cultural backgrounds, concern about confidentiality of personal information shared, embarrassment about discussing sensitive topics, and fear of being arrested or deported while attempting to access services. Further information about how to address program participation barriers is provided in Section 3.

## DEVELOPING AND USING PROGRAM MODELS

### What Are Program Models?

A *program model* (also called a *logic model*) is a visual representation of your goals and objectives (what your program seeks to achieve) and the corresponding program components (strategies, activities, and services) that you will employ to achieve them (Card et al., 2001). Your program model should reflect your target population's needs and assets, your agency's philosophy and resources, and research-based approaches to HIV prevention. Several examples of program models are provided in Figure 2–5.

## Program Model Uses

Developing a program model does not require a large investment of resources, but it offers many benefits. In particular, program modeling can help you and your stakeholders to:

- Develop or adapt a program to address local needs.
- Achieve consensus on, and commitment, to program design.
- Identify and address weaknesses in program design.
- Allocate resources across program components.
- Identify what program "success" would look like from process and outcome perspectives.
- Communicate with others (e.g., agency colleagues, Boards, community members, funders) about your program.

## Steps in Developing Culturally Competent Program Models

Once key stakeholders have agreed on a definition of the problem to be addressed in the community, decided whether to base the program on a formal theory, and identified culturally appropriate goals, objectives, and program components that address target population needs, the program model is relatively simple to construct. The target population description, goals, objectives, and programs components can be summarized in a table or diagram format such as the examples in Figure 2–5. It is helpful to draw arrows to show links between program components, objectives, and goals.

Once the links are drawn, it is important to assess the strength of the model. Examples of model strength criteria include (Kirby, 2004; Sedivy, 2000):

- **Needs and Assets:** To what extent does the model address HIV-related needs and assets of the target population, local community, and agency?
- **Cultural Factors**: How robustly are cultural factors influencing HIV risk addressed? Is the intervention consistent with local cultural norms?
- **Coherence**: Does the model present a coherent picture of the intervention?
- **Strength of Links**: How strong are links among program components, objectives, and goals?
- **Best Practices**: How robustly are characteristics common to effective program included in the program? Examples of such characteristics are provided in Table 2–5.
- **Consensus**: Is there consensus on the model among key stakeholders?

Tool 2–11: Program Model Development Worksheet can help you to construct and assess the strength of your program model.

Your program model should be revisited periodically—for example, once a year or when a funding cycles ends. Keeping your model up-to-date will help with subsequent program planning, implementation, and evaluation processes, and it will help ensure that a current model is always available to share with others.

**MODEL #1: HIV TESTING AND COUNSELING, EDUCATION, AND SKILLS-BUILDING INTERVENTION FOR INJECTION DRUG USERS**

*Target Population:*  | 500 men and women ages 18–35 of varied ethnicities who use injection drugs

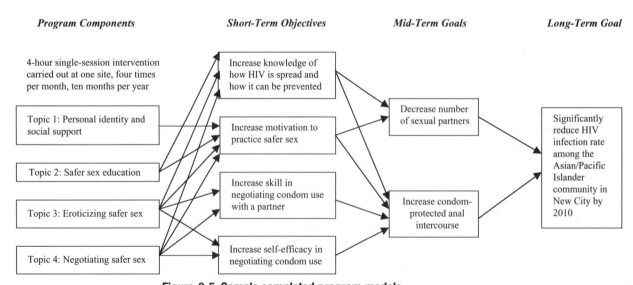

Figure 2-5  Sample completed program models.

**MODEL #3: GROUP EDUCATIONAL AND SKILLS-BUILDING INTERVENTION FOR AFRICAN-AMERICAN YOUNG WOMEN**

*Target Population:*   African-American young women ages 18–29

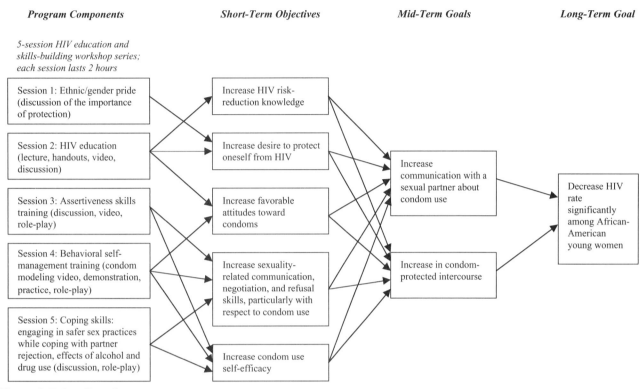

**Figure 2-5  (continued)**

## Making Your Model a Good Communication Tool

As was indicated earlier, your program model can help you communicate about your program with persons outside your department or agency. To make the model an effective communication tool, be sure to keep it simple. Including every detail about your program is not necessary—each box in the model should include just a brief phrase. In addition, avoid using technical terms or acronyms that are not likely to be known beyond your program staff, or provide a key at the bottom of the model that defines them. Finally, be sure to put a date on your model to make clear when it was last updated.

## REPLICATING EXISTING PROGRAMS VERSUS DEVELOPING NEW PROGRAMS

### What Is Replication?

*Replication* is the process of moving an intervention to a new site in a way that maintains fidelity (faithfulness) to its underlying theory, overarching goals, and principal components—but also permits adaptation to the new context (Backer, 2001; Kelly et al., 2000). A well-chosen, carefully planned program that is implemented with fidelity to its original developer's intent and design has a much greater likelihood of achieving positive outcomes. Because needs and resources differ from site to site, however, you should consider whether replicating an existing program, developing

| Characteristics Common to Effective HIV Prevention Programs

---

### COMMON CHARACTERISTICS OF BEHAVIORAL PREVENTION PROGRAMS*

Programs for HIV-positive and/or HIV-negative persons
- Are based on formal behavioral and/or social theories
- Build relevant sexual and/or drug-related risk reduction skills
- Are culturally tailored for their target population(s)

(CDC, 2001; Kelly & Kalichman, 2002; Kirby et al., 2006)

### *ADDITIONAL* COMMON CHARACTERISTICS OF BEHAVIORAL PREVENTION PROGRAMS FOR SPECIFIC POPULATIONS*

Programs for men who have sex with men (MSM)
- Incorporate multiple (i.e., four or more) delivery methods, such as counseling, group discussions, lectures, live demonstrations, and role plays
- Are delivered over multiple sessions spanning a minimum of three weeks

(Herbst et al., 2005)

Programs for women
- Emphasize gender influences (e.g., power imbalances)
- Are peer-led
- Involve multiple sessions

(DiClemente & Wingood, 1996; Exner et al., 1997; Mize et al., 2002)

Programs for people who inject drugs
- Provide equivalent content on sex- and drug-related HIV risk
- Include use of multiple theories and methods
- Include role modeling and social support enhancement

(Copenhaver et al., 2006; Des Jarlais & Semaan, 2005; van Empelen et al., 2003)

Programs for HIV-positive persons
- Focus on reduction of specific sexual risk behaviors
- Are delivered by health care providers or counselors on a one-on-one basis
- Are delivered in an intensive manner (i.e., over 20 hours of contact during 10 or more sessions)
- Are delivered in settings where HIV-positive persons receive routine services or medical care
- Address a myriad of issues related to mental health, medication adherence, and HIV risk behavior

(Crepaz et al., 2006)

HIV education curricula for youth
- Focus on specific behaviors that prevent HIV (e.g., abstaining from sex, using condoms)
- Include multiple activities to change specific risk and protective factors that affect the sexual behaviors
- Create a safe environment for youth
- Involve participants actively and help them personalize the information
- Employ activities that are appropriate for youths' age and sexual experience
- Cover topics in a logical sequence
- Secure at least minimal support from appropriate authorities (e.g., school principals, clinic directors)
- Select educators/facilitators with desired characteristics, train them, and provide ongoing monitoring and support

(Kirby et al., 2006)

---

* It should be noted that *not all effective programs* for particular populations have *all* of the indicated characteristics. Also, incorporation of these characteristics does *not* guarantee program effectiveness.

The following Web-based resources can help you to identify the most effective HIV prevention programs for adults and youth:

- The Centers for Disease Control and Prevention's (CDC) *Compendium of HIV Prevention Interventions with Evidence of Effectiveness*: http://www.cdc.gov/hiv/pubs/hivcompendium/hivcompendium.htm

- CDC's *Replicating Effective Programs Plus* Web site: http://www.cdc.gov/hiv/projects/rep/

- The *Diffusion of Effective Behavioral Interventions (DEBI)* Web site: http://www.effectiveinterventions.org/

- Sociometrics Corporation's *HIV/AIDS Prevention Program Archive (HAPPA)*: http://www.socio.com/happa.htm

- Sociometrics Corporation's *Program Archive on Sexuality, Health and Adolescence (PASHA):* http://www.socio.com/pasha.htm

- ETR Associates' *Resource Center for Adolescent Pregnancy Prevention (ReCAPP):* http://www.etr.org/recapp/

**Figure 2-6 Tip: Web-based information on programs with the strongest evidence of effectiveness.**

a new one, or creating a *hybrid* (i.e., using different elements of existing programs) will work best for your organization and target population (Castro et al., 2004; Gandelman & Reitmeijer, 2004).

Programs that have undergone outcome evaluation and shown positive effects should be replicated with fidelity to the *core program,* which may be defined as the basic content and design elements that are responsible for those effects (Kelly et al., 2000; Stanton et al., 2005). Defining the core program (which is discussed further later in this section) is particularly important when you are undertaking adaptation of an effective program, because it is crucial not to undermine the aspects of the program that made it work in the first place.

## Assessing Candidate Programs for Replication

In deciding whether and what to replicate, consider the following aspects of existing programs (Backer, 2001; Kelly, 2000; Solomon et al., 2006):

1. Similarity of the original target population to your target population—especially with respect to developmental level, HIV-risk level, and cultural factors that influence HIV risk.
2. Appropriateness of program goals, objectives, and program activities and materials for target population and community needs and norms.
3. Strength of evidence of the program's effectiveness in achieving its goals and objectives. (Credible information on the programs with the strongest evidence of effectiveness, based on rigorous evaluation studies, may be found on the Web sites shown in Figure 2–6.)
4. Incorporation of characteristics common to effective programs that have taken the same approach (e.g., an HIV education approach or an HIV counseling and testing approach).
5. Appropriateness for agency philosophy and resources (e.g., staffing, funding, facilities, time with target population).
6. Availability of replication kits or program materials.

## Deciding Whether and What to Replicate

If a candidate program is a good match on all selection criteria described above, then it is best to replicate it with few or no adaptations (Kirby, 2001). If no candidate program is a good match on all criteria, you should consider whether it would be best to replicate with adaptations or develop a new or hybrid program. In making a decision, consider the costs and benefits of each option, given your available resources. Examples of some specific questions to consider are:

■ Would replicating require you to make fundamental changes to program objectives and components or more surface-level changes to materials?
■ If you replicate with adaptations, would the original program developer be available to help with planning?
■ Do your funders favor replication with adaptations, or development of a new or hybrid program?
■ Which route would best meet the needs of your clients while fitting your resource constraints?

If you decide to replicate, you may have to choose from among several programs, none of which is an ideal match. In this situation, it is helpful to bear in mind that if a program has never undergone outcome evaluation, you cannot know whether it has had positive effects in any context. It is therefore usually best to select a program that has already been evaluated and shown positive results with at least one group, ideally a population that is very similar to your target population. If this is not possible, then the next best option is to select a program that has robustly incorporated characteristics common to effective programs that have taken a similar approach or been shown to be effective with a similar population (Kirby, 2001; National Campaign, 2006). Examples of these characteristics were shown in Table 2.5. Tool 2–12: Replication Decision-Making Worksheet can help you to decide whether and what to replicate.

## ADAPTING PROGRAMS

### What Is Adaptation?

*Adaptation* is the process of altering a program to reduce mismatches between that program and the new community in which is it to be implemented (Castro et al., 2004). As was indicated earlier, it is best to select a program for replication that has shown strong evidence of effectiveness, and to replicate it in a similar context with few or no changes (Kirby, 2001). Each new implementation setting, however, will differ from the original in some way. This creates the potential for a mismatch between the program's approach, content, delivery methods, or required staffing, and the new setting. Examples of sources of mismatch are shown in Table 2–6.

### Identifying the Core Program

In adapting an effective program for a new setting, it is important to retain fidelity (faithfulness) to the core program, those content and design elements that are responsible for the program's effectiveness. For effective programs, the core program can be identified by means of (Kelly et al., 2000; McKleroy et al., 2006; Solomon et al., 2006):

■ The formal theory (or theories) underlying the program. The goals, objectives, and program features that directly address the theory's tenets can be considered core components.
■ Program developers' and evaluators' experience with the program.
■ Research that tests the effects of different versions of the program and identifies which features (e.g., peer vs. adult leaders; number of contact hours) are crucial to achieving the desired outcomes.

Sources of Mismatch Between Existing Programs and New
Implementation Sites (Castro et al., 2004; Bernal et al., 1995;
Dévieux, et al., 2004)

| Source of Mismatch | Specific Examples |
|---|---|
| **Characteristics of clients** | ■ Developmental level<br>■ Level of behavioral risk<br>■ Cultural norms and values<br>■ Language background<br>■ Literacy level |
| **Characteristics of agencies** | ■ Philosophy<br>■ Staff credentials/expertise<br>■ Staff cultural competence<br>■ Available resources |
| **Characteristics of communities** | ■ Cultural norms and values<br>■ Laws, regulations, or policies (e.g., concerning needle exchange)<br>■ Infrastructure (e.g., transportation) |

## Using a Program Modeling Process to Adapt a Program

A program modeling process can facilitate the reduction of mismatches between an intervention and a new context (Solomon et al., 2006; Tortolero et al., 2005). It can also help you monitor the adapted program's fidelity to core program elements. To use a program modeling process to adapt a program, follow these steps.

1. Develop a program model for the original intervention (Tool 2–11: Program Model Development Worksheet can help with this process), or, if possible, obtain a model from the intervention's developer. If the original intervention was shown to be effective through an evaluation study, identify the core program elements, based on the methods indicated above, and mark them on the model.
2. Review the long-term goals first; then the mid-term and short-term objectives; then the program components. As you review each element, make edits to reduce mismatches with your context. If the original intervention was effective, do not delete or undermine any core program elements. For example, it is important to be aware reducing the length or intensity of an intervention that has demonstrated positive outcomes may make a program ineffective (Robin et al., 2004). If possible, discuss the potential effects of program changes with the program's original developer or evaluator.
3. Make sure that in the revised model, program components remain logically linked to objectives, and objectives to goals.
4. Subject the revised model to tests of program model strength (as discussed earlier). This includes, for example, ensuring that the revised model robustly incorporates characteristics common to effective programs that have taken similar approaches or been successful with similar populations. (Examples of these characteristics were shown in Table 2–5.)

## Ensuring Culturally Competent Adaptation

As in the case of other program planning activities, involving representatives of the target population in the adaptation process can help ensure that the adaptations are appropriate for and acceptable to the intended clients. In addition, it is important to keep in mind that program content, format, and materials may not be the only

## 2-4   Using Program Modeling to Adapt a Youth Sexual Risk Reduction Intervention

Susan Tortolero and her colleagues from the University of Texas Health Science Center and the University of Houston knew what they were looking for. They needed an effective youth sexual risk reduction program, one that they could adapt for use with higher-risk students attending alternative high schools in Texas (Tortolero et al., 2005). After investigating their options, they decided to adapt the *Safer Choices* program.

*Safer Choices* is a theory-based, youth-focused HIV, STI, and pregnancy prevention program. It was originally implemented and evaluated with ethnically diverse youth attending high schools in San Jose, CA and Houston, TX (Coyle et al., 1996; Coyle et al., 1999; Coyle et al., 2001). Over a 31-month period, schools running the program saw a number of successful results, including:

- Reduced frequency of sex without a condom.
- Reduced number of partners with whom students had unprotected sex.
- Increased use of effective contraception and condom use at last sex.

In fact, the *Safer Choices* program reduced one or more measures of sexual risk among all groups of youth involved in the study. It was especially effective with males, Hispanics, and youth who had already engaged in unprotected sex prior to the study and were thus at higher risk for HIV, other STIs, and pregnancy (Kirby et al., 2004).

In adapting *Safer Choices* for high-risk students in Texas, Tortolero and her colleagues thought about how they could preserve the effectiveness of the original program while making sure it was relevant and appropriate for their students. They decided to use a process called intervention mapping (IM). Similar to program modeling, IM involves the following nine steps:

1. *Conduct a needs assessment.* The team first conducted focus groups and interviews with alternative high school students, and reviewed relevant existing studies. These activities helped them better understand students' risk-taking behaviors and the factors shaping these behaviors. Two interesting findings from this research were that (a) girls reported dating older men and experiencing difficulties negotiating condom use with them; and (b) students reported that sex was often being used to obtain material possessions or achieve social status.

2. *Review behavioral outcomes.* The team then reviewed *Safer Choice*'s desired behavioral outcomes and made some changes to accommodate the needs of the new group. For example, because most of the new population was already sexually active, the original program goal of reducing the number of students who had sex during high school was changed. The new goal was to increase the number of students choosing not to have sex when they did not want to have sex.

3. *Specify "performance objectives."* The team also decided on specific behavioral skills ("performance objectives") students would need to learn for the behavioral outcomes to be achieved. For example, to help students learn how to avoid unwanted sex, they would need to learn how to avoid high-risk situations that might lead to sex, and to better communicate their relationship preferences and needs.

4. *Specify determinants of behavior.* The team identified the psychological, social, and other factors influencing behavior that were addressed by the *Safer Choices* program. They then modified these to fit the needs of the new population. In particular, they wanted to be sure the adapted program would address issues of power in relationships, gender role expectations, and students' attitudes and hopes about their future.

5. *Develop "learning objectives."* The team developed a table that identified the connections between each behavior they wanted to affect, factors shaping that behavior, and the related learning objectives that would need to be achieved. To define the learning objectives, the team asked questions like "What knowledge is needed to obtain a condom?" and "What skills are needed to communicate the intention to use a condom?" These learning objectives became the focus for reviewing and adapting program strategies.

6. *Select theory-based, practical methods and strategies.* The team reviewed the *Safer Choices* content and delivery formats. Would these be appropriate for and consistent with the revised program objectives? For example, the original *Safer Choices* program included the creation of peer resources. This task was deleted in the adapted program, since students at the alternative schools were not strongly connected to school peer groups. In addition, new activities on healthy versus unhealthy relationships were added to address power issues and gender role expectations. Journal writing and the use of a video were also added to address new learning objectives.

7. *Develop the revised program.* The revised learning objectives and their corresponding activities were grouped into a lesson sequence. New materials such as a video were developed as needed. A youth advisory board provided input on all aspects of curriculum development.

8. *Address adoption and implementation issues.* The alternative high school students had a high drop-out rate. As such, the program was adapted into a shorter but more intensive intervention. Also, given the target population's mistrust of the educational system, program facilitators (rather than teachers) whose ethnic backgrounds were similar to that of students were trained to deliver the program.

9. *Evaluate the program.* As of the preparation of this "Tale from the Field," rigorous evaluation of the adapted program is currently underway.

Is the adapted *Safer Choices 2* program developed by Tortolero and her colleagues "the same intervention" as the original *Safer Choices*? The answer to this question isn't clear-cut. When adaptation takes place, the line between what constitutes "the same" versus "different" programs may blur (Stanton et al., 2005). Nonetheless, the project team did use a thoughtful process for adapting the *Safer Choices* program by:

- Paying close attention to the theories underlying the original program and making sure the adapted program reflected these theories.
- Making certain that in their adapted program matrix, there were logical links between (a) the desired behavioral outcomes, (b) the factors shaping these behaviors, and (c) the proposed adapted activities.
- Involving a youth advisory board in the adaptation process.

Using these strategies helps increase the likelihood that the adapted program will also show positive effects.

A replication kit for the original *Safer Choices* program is available through Sociometrics' Program Archive on Sexuality, Health & Adolescence (PASHA)—see http://www.socio.com/srch/summary/pasha/passt21.htm.

aspects of the intervention that need adaptation. Participant recruitment or retention strategies that were used in the original program implementation may need to be altered to meet the needs of the new population and community context. Moreover, staff training content and procedures may need to be changed to ensure that program staff are properly prepared to implement the adapted program, as it has been planned, with the intended participants.

Tool 2–13: Adaptation Checklist provides a step-by-step guide to the systematic adaptation of effective programs (i.e., programs that have shown positive outcomes in at least one rigorous outcome evaluation study). Real-life examples of how effective programs have been adapted for different populations are provided in Tale 2–4 to 2–6.

## 2-5   Adapting a Secondary HIV Prevention Program for HIV+ Recovering Drug Abusers

Imagine the potential levels of stress and depression for men and women who are (a) recovering drug abusers, and (b) HIV+ and undergoing highly active antiretroviral therapy (HAART). What are the effects of such stress and depression? Do they lead people to engage in further risky behavior? Or to have trouble sticking to a treatment regimen? If so, how can secondary HIV prevention interventions help?

*Secondary HIV prevention programs* are designed to help support HIV-related preventive behavior among people who are already HIV+. This is the type of program that interested Jessy Dévieux and her colleagues at Florida International University's AIDS Prevention Program. Dévieux and her team wanted to better address the HIV prevention needs of a diverse population in Miami. The population, ages 18–60, included English-speaking Hispanic and black HIV+ males and females who were undergoing HAART (Dévieux et al., 2004). To address their complex needs, the team adapted a group-based cognitive behavioral stress management (CBSM) intervention for use with recovering drug abusers.

The original CBSM intervention emphasized skills training and stress reduction. Over the past decade, it has been developed for use with HIV+ populations to promote adherence to treatment, most recently HAART. Pilot data had shown that CBSM could produce clinical improvement in people's depression/distress levels, as well as their immune system functioning. When adapting the CBSM program for recovering drug abusers (RDAs), the research team wanted to ensure the program focused on the complex relationships between risky sexual behavior, substance use, and people's willingness to stick with their HAART treatment regimens. How could this be accomplished?

The program planning team first sought program adaptation feedback from multiple sources. These included: (a) focus groups representing the new client population; (b) in-depth interviews with persons with a recent history of drug dependency; (c) interviews with local service providers serving the target group; (d) insights from a local medical anthropologist who was familiar with the region and its RDA population; and (e) an ongoing review of related scientific literature. Through these efforts, the team was able to decide on three key cultural dimensions (Bernal et al., 1995) that the adapted program (CBSM-RDA) should address:

1. *Program staffing.* The team knew that the greater the similarity between clients and service providers in terms of cultural values and practices, the more likely the program would use content and processes that promoted positive behavioral change. The planning team decided that the program would be implemented by two-member facilitation teams, each made up of one black and one Hispanic, and one male and one female. In addition, one team member would be a professional therapist and the other a well-trained peer who was a recovered addict.
2. *Language.* The team also understood that interventions should take into account clients' language and the cultural meanings conveyed through that language. Although the CBSM-RDA (and the original CBSM) were developed for use with an English-speaking population, various language issues still needed to be addressed. For example, professional and popular terms (for things like body parts or drug equipment) differed, as did the vocabulary used by diverse ethnic groups. Target population members also differed in their ability to read terminology on visual materials.
3. A facilitator's manual was developed to help staff implement the program with fidelity to the core program components. The manual also:
   □ Provides facilitators with alternate (lay) vocabulary for all technical terms.
   □ Encourages facilitators to ask clients to explain "street" terms they use, so that these terms are clear to participants from other backgrounds.
   □ Uses gender-neutral terms such as "partner" (instead of "boyfriend" or "girlfriend") in activity scripts to help staff avoid assumptions about clients' sexual orientation.

3. *Cultural knowledge and social context.* Finally, the research team understood that many factors shape the ways people use the knowledge and skills promoted by an intervention. These factors include cultural values and beliefs, social supports, gender roles, and socioeconomic status. For example, in some ethnic groups, women may not feel free to insist openly and directly that a more powerful male partner use condoms. They may learn other strategies for negotiating condom use, such as "unspoken agreements" to make shared decisions in private, while maintaining a public appearance that the male is the decision maker. The program planning team designed activities that encouraged participants to develop, discuss, and practice culturally appropriate strategies for reducing risky behavior and increasing HAART adherence.

In adapting the intervention, the planning team didn't focus on the needs of just one or a few ethnic groups within the target population. Instead, they drew on the common experiences of all group members, representing diverse ethnicities, genders, and sexual orientations. These common experiences included feelings of hopelessness related to poverty and loss of power; stress related to AIDS progression (e.g., loss of work, increased medical costs, self-care difficulties, social isolation); and the difficulty of reducing risky behaviors in these situations. The team worked to develop a group-based intervention that would allow members to participate as equals and develop new social supports for recovering from drug abuse, experiencing HIV, and adhering to HAART.

As of the writing of this "Tale from the Field," an evaluation of the CBSM-RDA is in progress.

## TALE FROM THE FIELD

## 2-6 Adapting the Popular Opinion Leaders (POL) Program for Use at "Hustler" Bars

According to to one 1991 study of male prostitutes who have sex with men (*hustlers*) in Atlanta, a staggering 29% were HIV-positive (Elifson, 1991). Findings like this concerned staff at the Gay Men's Health Crisis (GMHC), a large community-based organization in New York City. GMHC staff decided that New York City "hustler bars" offered a promising location for implementing an adapted version of the *Popular Opinion Leaders* (POL) program (Miller, 2003).

The original POL program was designed by Jeff Kelly and colleagues at the Medical College of Wisconsin to reduce unprotected sex among male patrons of gay bars. POL uses *popular opinion leaders* (i.e., bar patrons that other patrons look up to) to deliver safer sex messages, supporting the idea that safer sex is the norm among respected and admired people. The POL program has shown promising results in lowering rates of unprotected

anal intercourse among bar patrons who have participated in the intervention (Kelly et al., 1991; Kelly et al., 1992; Kelly et al., 1997; see also Figure 2.3).

Staff at the GMHC felt the POL program would also work well with hustlers and their clients. In particular, it showed great potential for (Miller, 2003):

- Reaching the target population where they worked and socialized, instead of requiring them to seek services at an agency.
- Drawing on the bar-based hustler culture, where older, more experienced hustlers guide younger and inexperienced newcomers in the hustler world.
- Communicating messages tailored to the needs of hustlers and their clients, including men of diverse ethnic backgrounds.

- Being cost and resource effective—with the POL program, there is no need for a large agency space, a long program start-up, or credentialed staff, as just a few trained POL leaders can potentially change individual behaviors and group sexual behavior norms.

When Miller and her colleagues adapted the POL program for use at three New York City hustler bars, they followed several original intervention delivery steps, including: (1) training bartenders to identify natural leaders among patrons; (2) recruiting patrons who had been nominated by several bartenders as popular opinion leaders; and (3) training the opinion leaders to deliver safer sex messages to an agreed-upon number of peers. However, the team also adapted the content and delivery format of the original intervention to fit the new population:

- Role plays were rewritten to include situations that prostitutes might encounter, such as being offered more money for sex without a condom.
- Opinion leaders underwent training over a shorter timeframe to accommodate their unusual and varying schedules.
- Cash incentives were offered to compensate the opinion leaders for the time they spent in training.

Trained GMHC volunteers who were familiar with the hustler community were assigned to provide support to the opinion leaders and record their verbal reports of their activities. This ensured that opinion leaders with low literacy skills could participate in the intervention.

Was the adapted POL program successful in hustler bars? An evaluation of the intervention (which used similar procedures to that of the original POL evaluations) found large decreases in the proportion of men reporting paid, unprotected anal and oral sex in two of the three bars (Miller et al., 1998). The researchers also learned something interesting about the program's success in these two bars. It turned out that the opinion leaders in these bars felt a *sense of ownership of the intervention*. They participated more enthusiastically, developed a greater sense of connection among themselves, and expressed greater motivation to be effective than participants at the third bar in the study (Miller, 2003). Notably, opinion leaders at one of the two successful sites—frequented by Latino hustlers and men who identified as bisexual—told researchers they were surprised that anyone wanted to work with them. They felt most AIDS-related organizations did not care about them, and appreciated that someone believed in their potential to have a positive impact in their communities. From Miller's viewpoint, the "combination of commitment, enthusiasm, recognition, and ownership contributed to the intervention's effectiveness" in the hustler bar setting (Miller, 2003, p. 135).

For further information about the original POL, including how to obtain program materials and training in POL implementation, see http://www. effectiveinterventions.org/interventions/POL.cfm, a Web page of the Centers for Disease Control and Prevention-sponsored Diffusion of Effective Behavioral Interventions (DEBI) Project.

## RECRUITING AND TRAINING STAFF

*Program staff* can include agency employees, consultants, student interns, and volunteers. Their skill and dedication are essential to program success. It is therefore crucial that they be appropriately recruited and properly trained.

### Recruiting Staff

Before beginning to recruit candidates, it is helpful to prepare a brief (i.e., one- to two-page) announcement that describes your agency, program, and client background; the position duties and necessary qualifications; compensation; and application procedures and deadlines. Ideally, agency managers, current staff, and members of the program's target population should all provide input on staff characteristics that would be appealing to them. Tool 2–14: Template for Preparing a Position Announcement can help you to organize your announcement.

Once there is agreement on the position announcement, it can be circulated (in full or shortened form) by means of contacts at local agencies, hardcopy or Web postings in professional newsletters or Web sites, distribution of printed announcements at professional meetings, newspaper advertisements, and Web postings on local electronic community bulletin boards. It is particularly important to ensure that announcements are posted in places that are accessible to qualified applicants who are members of, or who have worked closely with, the program's target population.

## Assessing Candidates

You may wish to have a committee of current staff and members of your target population review all potential candidates. Their input can help ensure a good match with client needs and preferences. In assessing candidates, it is important to consider the following factors:

- The fit of candidate's knowledge, skills, experience, and attitudes for the position.
- The candidate's ability to work effectively with the program's target population and current staff.
- The candidate's commitment to the program's goals and methods.
- Opportunities for candidates to contribute to the program or agency beyond immediate position needs.

Tool 2–15: Template for Assessing Candidates can help you organize the information you collect about each candidate.

## Staff Training

Even the most experienced staff can benefit from additional training. It is important to ensure that both new and existing staff are properly trained in a variety of topics and skills, including (Adams et al., 2000; Gilbert, 2003a; OMH, 2001):

According to the U.S. Office of Minority Health's *National Standards for Culturally and Linguistically Appropriate Services in Health Care* (OMH, 2001), Standard 3, cultural competence training for staff should:

- **Be based on adult learning principles.** For example, adult learners are practical and problem-centered, so training should include examples that link theory to practice, as well as authentic activities that help participants to plan how they will apply the new information and skills on the job. In addition, training should build on participants' existing knowledge and help them recall what they already know that relates to the topic of learning. Information should also be delivered though multiple channels—for example, sound, written words, pictures—to keep learners interested and promote maximal absorption of concepts and skills (Best Practice Resources, n.d.; Yale University Library, 2001).
- **Tailor training objectives to trainees' functions and clients' needs.** Because there are so many potential training topics and approaches, but limited resources for providing training, it is important to determine which objectives are most important for trainees' current functions and clients' needs. Training activities and delivery methods should then be tailored to address these specific objectives.
- **Involve members of the client community in training program development.** The involvement of target population representatives from the earliest planning phases helps to ensure that staff trainings address the needs, cultural values, and views of the people that the agency serves.
- **Be ongoing.** In a climate of frequent staff turnover, ongoing staff training helps to ensure that both old and new staff members have common knowledge and practices. Ongoing training also helps to reinforce desirable knowledge, skills, and behaviors among staff.

**Figure 2-7 Tip: Cultural competence training for staff.**

1. Content and delivery methods of the program.
2. How to complete evaluation-related documentation (e.g., on program delivery and attendance).
3. Issues pertaining to cultural competence, including:
   ☐ Agency's or program's definition of cultural competence.
   ☐ How to be more aware of their own and others' cultural values.
   ☐ Effects of cultural factors on HIV risk and service utilization.
   ☐ Techniques for communicating more effectively with clients of different backgrounds (e.g., how to use interpreters appropriately).
   ☐ Strategies for resolving culturally based conflicts among staff and clients.
   ☐ Applicable regulations, policies, and procedures concerning clients' rights.

Some recommendations from the Office of Minority Health (OMH) concerning cultural competence training for staff are provided in Figure 2–7. Recent comprehensive lists of cultural competence staff training resources (e.g., models, guidebooks, videos, trainers, etc.) have been compiled by The California Endowment (e.g., see Gilbert et al., 2003a, 2000b, 2000c).

# REFERENCES

Adams, J., Terry, M. A., Rebchook, G. M., O'Donnell, L., Kelly, J. A., Leonard, N. R., et al. (2000). Orientation and training: Preparing agency administrators and staff to replicate an HIV prevention intervention. *AIDS Education and Prevention, 12*(Suppl A), 75–86.

Ajzen, I. (1988). *Attitudes, personality, and behavior.* Chicago: Dorsey.

Backer, T. E. (2001). *Finding the balance: Program fidelity and adaptation in substance abuse prevention: A state-of-the-art review.* Rockville, MD: Substance Abuse and Mental Health Services Administration, Center for Substance Abuse Prevention. Retrieved January 24, 2007, from http://modelprograms.samhsa.gov/pdfs/FindingBalance.pdf

Bandura, A. (1986). *Social foundations of thought and action: A social cognitive theory.* Englewood Cliffs, NJ: Prentice Hall.

Bandura, A. (1994). Social cognitive theory and the exercise of control over HIV infection. In R. J. DiClemente & J. Peterson (Eds.), *Preventing AIDS: Theories and methods of behavioral interventions* (pp. 25–29). New York: Plenum Publishing.

Bernal, G., Bonilla, J., & Bellido, C. (1995). Ecological validity and cultural sensitivity for outcome research: Issues for the cultural adaptation and development of psychosocial treatments with Hispanics. *Journal of Abnormal Child Psychology, 23*(1), 67–82.

Best Practice Resources. (n.d.). Principles of adult learning [adapted from John Goodlad]. Retrieved May 29, 2007, from http://www.teachermentors.com/RSOD%20Site/StaffDev/adultLrng.HTML

Brach, C., & Fraser, I. (2000). Can cultural competency reduce racial and ethnic health disparities? A review and conceptual model. *Medical Care Research and Review, 57*(1), 181–217.

Brettle, R. P. (1991). HIV and harm reduction for injection drug users. *AIDS, 5*(2), 125–136.

Brindis, C., & Davis, L. (1998). *Improving contraceptive access for teens. (Communities responding to the challenge of adolescent pregnancy prevention, Vol. IV).* Washington, DC: Advocates for Youth. Retrieved August 2, 2005, from http://www.advoratesforyouth.org/publications/communitiesresponding4.pdf

Butterfoss, F. D., Goodman, R. M., & Wandersman, A. (1996). Community coalitions for prevention and health promotion: Factors predicting satisfaction, participation, and planning. *Health Education Quarterly, 23*(1), 65–79.

Card, J. J., Brindis, C., Peterson, J. L., & Niego, S. (2001). *Guidebook: Evaluating teen pregnancy prevention programs* (2nd ed.). Los Altos, CA: Sociometrics Corporation.

Carrillo, J. E., Green, A. R., & Betancourt, J. R. (1999). Cross-cultural primary care: A patient-based approach. *Annals of Internal Medicine, 130*(10), 829–834.

Castro, F. G., Barrera, M., Jr., & Martinez, C. R., Jr. (2004). The cultural adaptation of prevention interventions: Resolving tensions between fidelity and fit. *Prevention Science, 5*(1), 41–45.

Catania, J. A., Kegeles, S. M., & Coates, T. J. (1990). Towards an understanding of risk behavior: An AIDS risk reduction model (AARM). *Health Education Quarterly, 17*(1), 53–72.

Centers for Disease Control and Prevention (CDC). (2001). *Compendium of HIV prevention interventions with evidence of success.* Atlanta, GA: CDC. Retrieved October 13, 2004, from http://www.cdc.gov/hiv/pubs/hivcompendium/hivcompendium.htm

Child Welfare League of America. (1993). *Cultural competence self-assessment instrument*. Washington, DC: Child Welfare League of America.

Choi, K. H., Lew, S., Vittinghoff, E., Catania, J. A., Barrett, D. C., & Coates, T. J. (1996). The efficacy of brief group counseling in HIV risk reduction among homosexual Asian and Pacific Islander men. *AIDS, 10*(1), 81–87.

Connell, R. W. (1987). *Gender and power*. Stanford, CA: Stanford University Press.

Copenhaver, M. M., Johnson, B. T., Lee, I.-C., Harman, J. J., Carey, M. P., & the SHARP Research Team. (2006). Behavioral HIV risk reduction among people who inject drugs: Meta-analytic evidence of efficacy. *Journal of Substance Abuse Treatment, 31*(2), 163–171.

Coyle, K., Basen-Engquist, K., Kirby, D., Parcel, G., Banspach, S., Collins, J., et al. (2001). Safer Choices: Reducing teen pregnancy, HIV, and STDs. *Public Health Reports, 116*(Suppl. 1), 82–93.

Coyle, K., Basen-Engquist, K., Kirby, D., Parcel, G., Banspach, S., Harrist, R., et al. (1999). Short-term impact of Safer Choices: A multicomponent, school-based HIV, other STD, and pregnancy prevention program. *Journal of School Health, 69*(5), 181–188.

Coyle, K., Kirby, D., Parcel, G., Basen-Engquist, K., Banspach, S., Rugg, D., et al. (1996). Safer Choices: A multicomponent school-based HIV/STD and pregnancy prevention program for adolescents. *Journal of School Health, 66*(3), 89–94.

Crepaz, N., Lyles, C. M., Wolitski, R. J., Passin, W. F., Rama, S. M., Herbst, J. H., et al. & the HIV Prevention Research Synthesis (PRS) Team. (2006). Do prevention interventions reduce HIV risk behaviours among people living with HIV? A meta-analytic review of controlled trials. *AIDS, 20*(2), 143–157.

Des Jarlais, D. C., & Semaan, S. (2005). Interventions to reduce the sexual risk behaviour of injecting drug users. *International Journal of Drug Policy, 16*(Suppl), S58–S66.

Dévieux, J. G., Malow, R. M., Rosenberg, R., & Dyer, J. G. (2004). Context and common ground: Cultural adaptation of an intervention for minority HIV-infected individuals. *Journal of Cultural Diversity, 11*(2), 49–57.

DiClemente, R. J., & Wingood, G. M. (1995). A randomized controlled trial of an HIV sexual risk-reduction intervention for African-American women. *Journal of the American Medical Association, 274*(16), 1271–1276.

DiClemente, R. J., Wingood, G. M., Harrington, K. F., Lang, D. L., Davies, S. L., Hook, E. W., III, et al. (2004). Efficacy of an HIV prevention intervention for African American adolescent girls. *Journal of the American Medical Association, 292*(2), 171–179.

Elifson, K. W., Boles, J., & Sweat, M. (1991, November). *Risk factors associated with HIV-seroprevalence among male prostitutes*. Paper presented at the 119th Annual Meeting of the American Public Health Association, Atlanta, GA.

Exner, T. M., Seal, D. W., & Ehrhardt, A. A. (1997). A review of HIV interventions for at-risk women. *AIDS and Behavior, 1*(2), 93–124.

Fishbein, M., & Ajzen, I. (1975). *Belief, attitude, intention, and behavior: An introduction to theory and research*. Reading, MA: Addison Wesley.

Fishbein, M., Triandis, H. C., Kanfer, F. H., Becker, M., Middlestadt, S. E., & Eichler, A. (2001). Factors influencing behavior and behavior change. In A. Baum, T. A. Revenson, & J. E. Singer (Eds.), *Handbook of health psychology* (pp. 3–17). Mahwah, NJ: Lawrence Erlbaum Associates.

Fisher, J. D., & Fisher, W. A. (1992). Changing AIDS-risk behavior. *Psychological Bulletin, 111*(3), 455–474.

The Florida Department of Health. (2004). Community health status and improvement planning terminology. Retrieved August 1, 2005, from http://www.doh.state.fl.us/planning_eval/CHAI/Resources/FieldGuide/6CommHealthStatus/CHSATerminology.htm

Fortier, J. P., Convissor, R., & Pacheco, G. (1999). *Assuring cultural competence in health care: Recommendations for national standards and an outcomes-focused research agenda*. Washington, DC: Department of Health and Human Services and Resources for Cross Cultural Health Care.

Gandelman, A., & Reitmeijer, C. A. (2004). Translation, adaptation, and synthesis of interventions for persons living with HIV: Lessons from previous HIV prevention interventions. *Journal of Acquired Immune Deficiency Syndromes, 37*(Suppl 2), S126–S129.

Gilbert, M. J. (Ed.). (2003a). *A manager's guide to cultural competence education for health care professionals*. Woodlands, CA: The California Endowment. Retrieved May 12, 2005, from http://www.calendow.org/reference/publications/pdf/cultural/TCE0217-2003_A_Managers_Gui.pdf

Gilbert, M. J. (Ed.). (2003b). *Principles and recommended standards for cultural competence education of health care professionals*. Woodlands, CA: The California Endowment. Retrieved January 16, 2006, from http://www.calendow.org/reference/publications/pdf/cultural/TCE0215-2003_Principles_and.pdf

Gilbert, M. J. (Ed.). (2003c). *Resources in cultural competence education for health care professionals*. Woodlands, CA: The California Endowment. Retrieved January 16, 2006, from http://www.calendow.org/reference/publications/pdf/cultural/TCE0218-2003_Resources_in_C.pdf

Hamdallah, M., Vargo, S., & Herrera, J. (2006). The VOICES/VOCES success story: Effective strategies for training, technical assistance and community-based organization implementation. *AIDS Education and Prevention*, *18*(4 Suppl A), 171–183.

Harshbarger, C., Simmons, G., Coelho, H., Sloop, K., & Collins, C. (2006). An empirical assessment of implementation, adaptation, and tailoring: The evaluation of CDC's national diffusion of VOICES/VOCES. *AIDS Prevention and Education*, *18* (Suppl A), 184–197.

Herbst, J. H., Sherba, R. T., Crepaz, N., DeLuca, J. B., Zohrabyan, L., Stall, R. D., et al. & the HIV/AIDS Prevention Research Synthesis (PRS) Team. (2005). A meta-analytic review of behavioral interventions for reducing sexual risk behavior of men who have sex with men. *Journal of Acquired Immune Deficiency Syndromes*, *39*(3), 228–241.

Herlocher, T., Hoff, C., & DeCarlo, P. (1996). *Can theory help in HIV prevention?* Center for AIDS Prevention Studies (CAPS), University of California San Francisco. Retrieved August 1, 2005, from http://www.hivpositive.com/f-HIVyou/2-Prevention/theorytext.html

Kalichman, S. C. (1998). *Preventing AIDS: A sourcebook for behavioral interventions*. Mahwah, NJ: Lawrence Erlbaum Associates.

Kelly, J. A., Heckman, T. G., Stevenson, L. Y., Williams, P. N., Ertl, T., Hays, R. B., et al. (2000). Transfer of research-based HIV prevention interventions to community service providers: Fidelity and adaptation. *AIDS Education and Prevention*, *12*(Suppl A), 87–98.

Kelly, J. A., & Kalichman, S. C. (2002). Behavioral research in HIV/AIDS primary and secondary prevention: Recent advances and future directions. *Journal of Consulting and Clinical Psychology*, *70*(3), 626–639.

Kelly, J. A., Murphy, D. A., Sikkema, K. J., McAuliffe, T. L., Roffman, R. A., Solomon, L. J., et al. & The Community HIV Prevention Research Collaborative. (1997). Randomised, controlled, community-level HIV-prevention intervention for sexual-risk behaviour among homosexual men in US cities. *Lancet*, *350*(9090), 1500–1505.

Kelly, J. A., St. Lawrence, J. S., Diaz, Y. E., Stevenson, L. Y., Hauth, A. C., Kalichman, S. C., et al. (1991). HIV risk behavior reduction following intervention with key opinion leaders of population: An experimental analysis. *American Journal of Public Health*, *81*(2), 1483–1489.

Kelly, J. A., St. Lawrence, J. S., Stevenson, L. Y., Hauth, A. C., Kalichman, S. C., Diaz, Y. E., et al. (1992). Community AIDS/HIV risk reduction: The effects of endorsements by popular people in three cities. *American Journal of Public Health*, *82*(11), 1483–1489.

Kennedy, M. G., Mizuno, Y., Hoffman, R., Baume, C., & Strand, J. (2000). The effect of tailoring a model HIV prevention program for local adolescent target audiences. *AIDS Education and Prevention*, *12*(3), 225–238.

Kirby, D. (2001). *Emerging answers: Research findings on programs to reduce teen pregnancy*. Washington, DC: National Campaign to Prevent Teen Pregnancy.

Kirby, D. (2002). Effective approaches to reducing adolescent unprotected sex, pregnancy, and childbearing. *The Journal of Sex Research*, *39*(1), 51–57.

Kirby, D. (2004). BDI logic models: A useful tool for designing, strengthening, and evaluating programs to reduce adolescent sexual risk-taking, pregnancy, HIV, and other STDs. Retrieved July 3, 2005, from http://www.etr.org/recapp/BDILOGICMODEL20030924.pdf

Kirby, D. B., Baumler, E., Coyle, K. K., Basen-Engquist, K., Parcel, G. S., Harrist, R., et al. (2004). The "Safer Choices" intervention: Its impact on the sexual behaviors of different subgroups of high school students. *Journal of Adolescent Health*, *35*(6), 442–452.

Kirby, D., Laris, B. A., & Rolleri, L. (2006). *Sex and HIV education programs for youth: Their impact and important characteristics*. Washington, DC: Family Health International. Retrieved March 18, 2007, from http://www.etr.org/recapp/programs/SexHIVedProgs.pdf

Lauby, J. L., Smith, P. J., Stark, M., Person, B., & Adams, J. (2000). A community-level prevention intervention for inner city women: Results of the Women and Infants Demonstration Projects. *American Journal of Public Health*, *90*(2), 216–222.

McKleroy, V. S., Galbraith, J. S., Cummings, B., Jones, P., Harshbarger, C., Collins, C., et al. (2006). Adapting evidence-based behavioral interventions for new settings and target populations. *AIDS Prevention and Education*, *18*(Suppl A), 59–73.

Miller, R. L. (2003). Adapting an evidence-based intervention: Tales of the Hustler Project. *AIDS Education and Prevention*, *15*(Suppl A), 127–138.

Miller, R. L., Klotz, D., & Eckholdt, H. M. (1998). HIV prevention with male prostitutes and patrons of hustler bars: replication of an HIV prevention intervention. *American Journal of Community Psychology*, *26*(1), 97–131.

Mize, S. J. S., Robinson, B. E., Bockting, W. O., & Scheltema, K. E. (2002). Meta-analysis of the effectiveness of HIV prevention interventions for women. *AIDS Care*, *14*(2), 163–180.

National Campaign to Prevent Teen Pregnancy. (2006). *What works: Curriculum-based programs that prevent teen pregnancy*. Washington, DC: National Campaign to Prevent Teen Pregnancy. Retrieved June 30, 2007, from http://www.teenpregnancy.org/product/pdf/10-5_2006_18_39_59What_Works.pdf

National Cancer Institute. (2005). *Theory at a glance: A guide for health promotion practice* (2nd ed.). NIH Publication No. 05–3896. U.S. Department of Health and Human Services, National Institutes of Health. Retrieved May 7, 2006, from http://www.cancer.gov/PDF/481f5d53- 63df-41bc-bfaf-5aa48ee1da4d/TAAG3.pdf

O'Donnell, C. R., O'Donnell, L., San Doval, A., Duran, R., & Labes, K. (1998). Reductions in STD infections subsequent to an STD clinic visit: Using video-based patient education to supplement provider interactions. *Sexually Transmitted Diseases*, *25*(3), 161–168.

O'Donnell, L., San Doval, A., Duran, R., & O'Donnell, C. R. (1995). The effectiveness of video-based interventions in promoting condom acquisition among STD clinic patients. *Sexually Transmitted Diseases*, *22*(2), 97–103.

O'Donnell, L., San Doval, A., Vornfett, R., & DeJong, W. (1994). Reducing AIDS and other STDs among inner-city Hispanics: The use of qualitative research in the development of video-based patient education. *AIDS Education and Prevention*, *6*(2), 140–153.

Office of Minority Health (OMH), U.S. Department of Health and Human Services. (2001). *National standards for culturally and linguistically appropriate services in health care: Final report*. Washington, DC: OMH. Retrieved January 16, 2006, from http://www.omhrc.gov/assets/pdf/checked/finalreport.pdf

Pedlow, C. T., & Carey, M. P. (2004). Developmentally appropriate sexual risk reduction interventions for adolescents: Rationale, review of interventions, and recommendations for research and practice. *Annals of Behavioral Medicine*, *27*(3), 172–184.

Peterson, J. L., Coates, T. J., Catania, J., Hauch, W. W., Acree, M., Daigle, D., et al. (1996). Evaluation of an HIV risk reduction intervention among African-American homosexual and bisexual men. *AIDS*, *10*(3), 319–325.

Porche, D. J., & Swayzer, R. (2003). HIV prevention: A review of interventions. *Journal of the Association of Nurses in AIDS Care*, *14*(1), 79–81.

Prochaska, J. O., DiClemente, C. C., & Norcross, J. C. (1992). In search of how people change: Applications to addictive behaviors. *American Psychologist*, *47*(9), 1102–1114.

Robin, L., Dittus, P., Whitaker, D., Crosby, R., Ethier, K., Mezoff, J., et al. (2004). Behavioral interventions to reduce incidence of HIV, STD, and pregnancy among adolescents: A decade in review. *Journal of Adolescent Health*, *34*(1), 3–26.

Rogers, E. M. (1983). *Diffusion of innovations* (3rd ed.). New York: The Free Press.

Rosenstock, M., Strecher, V., & Becker, M. (1994). The health belief model and HIV risk behavior change. In R. DiClemente & J. Peterson (Eds.), *Preventing AIDS: Theories, methods, and behavioral interventions* (pp. 5–24). New York: Plenum.

Scott, K. D., Gilliam, A., & Braxton, K. (2005). Culturally competent HIV prevention strategies for women of color in the United States. *Health Care for Women International*, *26*(1), 17–45.

Sedivy, V. (2000). *Is your program ready to evaluate its effectiveness? A guide to program assessment*. Los Altos, CA: Sociometrics Corporation and Washington, DC: National Organization on Adolescent Pregnancy, Parenting and Prevention (now called Healthy Teen Network).

Siegal, H. A., Falck, R. S., Carlson, R. G., & Wang, J. (1995). Reducing HIV needle risk behavior among injection-drug users in the Midwest: An evaluation of the efficacy of standard and enhanced interventions. *AIDS Education and Prevention*, *7*(4), 308–319.

Solomon, J., Card, J. J., & Malow, R. M. (2006). Adapting efficacious interventions: Advancing translational research in HIV prevention. *Evaluation and the Health Professions*, *29*(2), 162–194.

Somerville, G. G., Diaz, S., Davis, S., Coleman, K. D., & Taveras, S. (2006). Adapting the popular opinion leader intervention for Latino young migrant men who have sex with men. *AIDS Education and Prevention*, *18*(4 Suppl A), 137–148.

Stanton, B., Guo, J., Cottrell, L., Galbraith, J., Li, A., Gibson, C., et al. (2005). The complex business of adapting effective interventions to new populations: An urban to rural transfer. *Journal of Adolescent Health*, *37*(2), 163.e17–26.

Tortolero, S. R., Markham, C. M., Parcel, G. S., Peters, R. J., Jr., Escobar-Chaves, S. L., Basen-Engquist, K., et al. (2005). Using intervention mapping to adapt an effective HIV, sexually transmitted disease, and pregnancy prevention program for high-risk minority youth. *Health Promotion Practice*, *6*(3), 286–298.

van Empelen, P., Kok, G., van Kesteren, N. M. C., van den Borne, B., Bos, A. E. R., & Schaalma, H. P. (2003). Effective methods to change sex-risk among drug users: A review of psychosocial interventions. *Social Science & Medicine*, *57*(9), 1593–1608.

Vinh-Thomas, P., Bunch, M. M., & Card, J. J. (2003). A research-based tool for identifying and strengthening culturally competent and evaluation-ready HIV/AIDS prevention programs. *AIDS Education and Prevention*, *15*(6), 481–498.

Wingood, G. M., & DiClemente, R. J. (1996). HIV sexual risk reduction interventions for women: A review. *American Journal of Preventive Medicine*, *12*(3), 209–217.

Wingood, G. M., & DiClemente, R. J. (2000). Application of the theory of gender and power to examine HIV-related exposures, risk factors, and effective interventions for women. *Health Education & Behavior, 27*(5), 539–565.

Wingood, G. M., & DiClemente, R. J. (2006). Enhancing adoption of evidence-based HIV interventions: Promotion of a suite of HIV prevention interventions for African American women. *AIDS Education and Prevention, 18*(4 Suppl A), 161–170.

Wingood, G. M., DiClemente, R. J., Mikhail, I., Lang, D. L., McCree, D. H., Davies, S. L., et al. (2004). A randomized controlled trial to reduce HIV transmission risk behaviors and sexually transmitted diseases among women living with HIV: The WiLLOW Program. *Journal of Acquired Immune Deficiency Syndromes, 37*(Suppl 2), 58–67.

Wodak, A., & Cooney, A. (2006). Do needle syringe programs reduce HIV infection among injecting drug users: A comprehensive review of the international evidence. *Substance Use & Misuse, 41*(6–7), 777–813.

Yale University Library. (2001). Staff training & organizational development: Principles of adult learning. Retrieved May 29, 2007, from http://www.library.yale.edu/training/stod/principles.html

## Tool 2-1 Who Can Help With Community Needs and Assets Assessment?[1]

Working with local residents and other agencies can make your needs and assets (N&A) assessment a more manageable project—and one that better addresses the cultural needs of the populations you serve. Use the table below to list potential collaborators (e.g., other service agencies, consultants, community leaders, community volunteers, student interns from a local university) who may be able to assist in designing the assessment, collecting the data, or analyzing the results. In the far right column of the table, be sure to specify the kinds of assistance that your collaborators might provide.

To fill in the table below on your computer (using the file on the CD-ROM), click on the gray shaded area in the box you would like to type in. (Note that the gray shading will not appear in printouts of this document.) Alternately, you may photocopy this tool (for your own use only) and complete it by hand or typewriter.

| Name of Individual and/or Organization | Contact Information | Interest or Expertise | Possible N&A Assessment Task(s) (e.g., serving on N&A planning committee; organizing community forum event; etc.) |
|---|---|---|---|
| | | | |
| | | | |
| | | | |
| | | | |
| | | | |
| | | | |

---

[1] Adapted from Card, J. J., Brindis, C., Peterson, J. L., & Niego, S. (2001). *Guidebook: Evaluating teen pregnancy prevention programs* (2nd ed., Exercise 4.1). Los Altos, CA: Sociometrics Corporation.

# Tool 2-2 Sample Questions for a Needs and Assets Assessment[1]

Below are some sample needs and assets research questions. Place an "x" in the square box (□) next to the items that are of greatest relevance to your community or agency. (To do this on your computer—using the file on your CD-ROM—use your cursor to click on the box. To remove an "x" from a box, click on the box again.)

Use the blank "Additional questions" lines to write in other questions that are important to address. To do this on your computer, place your cursor on the gray-shaded area before beginning to type. (Note that the gray shading will not appear in printouts of this document.)

## I. Population Profile

### A. Demographic Characteristics

□ How many individuals live in the target community, by age, ethnic group, and language background?

□ What is the incidence of poverty in the community? Among the specific target population you are seeking to serve?

□ What is the incidence of school dropout in the community? Among the specific target population you are seeking to serve?

□ What is the incidence of unemployment in the community? Among the specific target population you are seeking to serve?

□ How many individuals are homeless? Among the specific target population you are seeking to serve?

□ *Additional question:*

□ *Additional question:*

### B. STI and HIV/AIDS Profile

□ How many <u>cases</u> of STIs, HIV infection, and AIDS are there in your community? Among the specific target population you are seeking to serve?

□ What are the <u>rates</u> of STIs, HIV infection, and AIDS in your community? Among the specific target population you are seeking to serve?

□ Among which subpopulation(s) are rates of STIs, HIV infection, and AIDS the highest? Among which are rates most increasing?

□ *Additional question:*

□ *Additional question:*

### C. Risk Behaviors and Circumstances

□ What types of sexual risk-taking behavior are most prevalent in the community (e.g., multiple partners, unprotected vaginal sex, unprotected anal sex, etc.)? Among the specific target population you are seeking to serve?

□ How many people in the community abuse alcohol or other drugs, including injection drugs? Among the specific target population you are seeking to serve?

□ What is the incidence of interpersonal violence (e.g., gang violence, relationship violence, child abuse) in the community? Among the specific target population you are seeking to serve?

□ *Additional question:*

□ *Additional question:*

---

[1] Adapted from Card, J. J., Brindis, C., Peterson, J. L., & Niego, S. (2001). *Guidebook: Evaluating teen pregnancy prevention programs* (2nd ed., Exercise 4.2). Los Altos, CA: Sociometrics Corporation.

### D. Access to Health Services

☐ How many people in the community have health insurance? Among the specific target population you are seeking to serve?

☐ For those in the community who do not have health insurance, how many have access to free or low-cost health services? Among the specific target population you are seeking to serve?

☐ *Additional question:*

☐ *Additional question:*

## II. Community Norms and Environment

### A. Community Values and Attitudes

☐ What knowledge, attitudes, and beliefs do community members have about HIV and AIDS?

☐ What knowledge, attitudes, and beliefs do community members have about the sexual and drug-related behaviors that lead to HIV infection?

☐ What knowledge, attitudes, and beliefs do community members have about interventions that can prevent the spread of HIV?

☐ What knowledge, attitudes, beliefs, and skills would need to be strengthened to help prevent the spread of HIV?

☐ What cultural factors constitute barriers or facilitators to preventing HIV?
    ☐ Attitudes toward talking with children or parents about sex?
    ☐ Gender roles and unequal power distribution in sexual relationships?
    ☐ Shame or stigma associated with homosexuality?
    ☐ Others?

☐ *Additional question:*

☐ *Additional question:*

### B. Policies

☐ What laws, regulations, and policies govern access to confidential HIV testing and counseling services for youth and adults (e.g., in clinics, schools, community organizations, correctional facilities, etc.)?

☐ What laws and policies govern access to other sexual and reproductive health services for youth and adults (e.g., in clinics, schools, community organizations, correctional facilities, etc.)?

☐ What laws and policies govern access to needle exchange, drug treatment, and other drug abuse-related services for youth and adults (e.g., in clinics, schools, community organizations, correctional facilities, etc.)?

☐ *Additional question:*

☐ *Additional question:*

## III. Resources

### A. Current HIV Prevention Programs

☐ What HIV prevention–related programs are already available in the community?
    ☐ Who offers these programs?
    ☐ What strategies to they use (e.g., HIV education, testing and counseling, media campaign, needle exchange)?
    ☐ What populations do they serve?
    ☐ What resources do they require?
    ☐ What challenges have they faced, and how have they addressed them?
    ☐ *Additional question:*
    ☐ *Additional question:*

☐ What barriers exist to clients' accessing HIV prevention services?
  ☐ What logistical barriers exist (e.g., transportation, scheduling, cost, availability of interpreting services), and how could they best be addressed?
  ☐ What perceived barriers exist (e.g., embarrassment about the topic, concerns about confidentiality issues, discomfort with staff of different cultural backgrounds), and how could they best be addressed?
  ☐ *Additional question:*
  ☐ *Additional question:*

## B. Effective Programs

☐ Nationwide, what HIV prevention programs have shown the strongest evidence of effectiveness?
  ☐ What approaches have they taken?
  ☐ What populations have they been shown to be effective with?
  ☐ What characteristics do they have in common?
  ☐ How appropriate would they be for use in your community and with your clients?

## C. Funding Opportunities

☐ What funding opportunities are available for HIV prevention programming in the community?
  ☐ Federal, state, and local government-sponsored opportunities?
  ☐ Private foundation opportunities?
  ☐ Corporate giving program opportunities?
  ☐ Grants from other private organizations (e.g., Rotary Club, religious institutions)
  ☐ Others?

☐ What funding opportunities would your agency be eligible to apply for?

☐ *Additional question:*

☐ *Additional question:*

## D. Other Sources of Assistance

☐ What other service organizations might your organization be able to collaborate with to plan, implement, or evaluate an HIV prevention program?

☐ What sources of volunteer assistance might you find in the community?
  ☐ Religious organizations
  ☐ Youth groups
  ☐ Private organizations (e.g., Rotary Club)
  ☐ Student interns from local colleges or universities
  ☐ Corporate volunteer programs

☐ *Additional question:*

☐ *Additional question:*

## E. Other

☐ *Additional question:*

☐ *Additional question:*

☐ *Additional question:*

## Tool 2-3 What Questions Do We Want Our Needs and Assets Assessment to Answer?[1]

Think about the kinds of questions you would like your assessment to address. You may wish to refer to the sample questions in Tool 2–2: Sample Questions for a Needs and Assets Assessment. Arrange your questions in priority order. Below are some prompts to help you begin.

To type directly into the tables below (using the file on the CD-ROM), click on the gray-shaded area in the box you would like to type in. (Note that the gray shading will not appear in printouts of this document.) Alternately, you may photocopy this tool (for your use only) and complete it by hand or typewriter.

A. High-priority questions about community **demographic characteristics**:

| |
|---|
| 1. |
| 2. |
| 3. |

B. High-priority questions about community **STI and HIV/AIDS rates**:

| |
|---|
| 1. |
| 2. |
| 3. |

C. High-priority questions about **key risk behaviors** in our community:

| |
|---|
| 1. |
| 2. |
| 3. |

D. High-priority questions about community **access to health services**:

| |
|---|
| 1. |
| 2. |
| 3. |

---

[1] Adapted from Card, J. J., Brindis, C., Peterson, J. L., & Niego, S. (2001). *Guidebook: Evaluating teen pregnancy prevention programs* (2nd ed., Exercise 4.3). Los Altos, CA: Sociometrics Corporation.

E. High-priority questions about community **values and attitudes**:

| |
|---|
| 1. |
| 2. |
| 3. |

F. High-priority questions about **policies** that affect our community:

| |
|---|
| 1. |
| 2. |
| 3. |

G. High-priority questions about **existing HIV prevention programs** in our community:

| |
|---|
| 1. |
| 2. |
| 3. |

H. High-priority questions about **effective HIV prevention programs**:

| |
|---|
| 1. |
| 2. |
| 3. |

I. High-priority questions about **funding opportunities** in our community:

| |
|---|
| 1. |
| 2. |
| 3. |

J. High-priority questions about other community sources of **program-related assistance**:

| |
|---|
| 1. |
| 2. |
| 3. |

K. Our **other** high-priority questions:

| |
|---|
| 1. |
| 2. |
| 3. |

# Tool 2-4 Sources of Needs and Assets Data

There are many potential sources of needs and assets data and information. Some examples are listed below.

| Type of Data | Examples of Existing Sources Outside Your Agency | Sources That Can Be Generated by Your Agency |
|---|---|---|
| Demographic characteristics | ■ U.S. Census<br>http://www.census.gov/ | ■ Your client registration or intake forms |
| STI and HIV/AIDS incidence and prevalence rates | ■ Centers for Disease Control and Prevention (CDC)<br>*HIV/AIDS Surveillance Reports*<br>http://www.cdc.gov/hiv/stats/hasrlink.htm<br>■ CDC<br>*STD Surveillance Reports*<br>http://www.cdc.gov/nchstp/dstd/Stats_Trends/Stats_and_Trends.htm<br>■ CDC's National Center for Health Statistics (NCHS)<br>*Fast Stats AIDS/HIV*<br>http://www.cdc.gov/nchs/fastats/aids-hiv.htm<br>■ Alan Guttmacher Institute<br>http://www.agi-usa.org/sections/youth.html<br>■ Kaiser Family Foundation<br>http://www.kaiserfamilyfoundation.org/ | ■ Your clients' medical records (if you have access to them) |
| Sexual and drug-related behaviors and experiences | ■ CDC<br>*Behavioral Risk Factor Surveillance System*<br>http://www.cdc.gov/brfss/index.htm<br>■ CDC<br>*Youth Risk Behavior Surveillance System*<br>http://www.cdc.gov/HealthyYouth/yrbs/index.htm<br>■ Your state or local public health department may also have local Behavior Risk Factor Survey or Youth Risk Behavior Survey data<br>■ Local universities, foundations, and other public or private agencies may also produce reports that contain local data | ■ Surveys of clients or community members<br>■ Focus group with clients or community members<br>■ Interviews with community leaders |
| Health service access | ■ CDC's National Center for Health Statistics<br>National Health Interview Survey<br>http://www.cdc.gov/nchs/nhis.htm<br>■ Local universities, foundations, and public or private health and social service agencies may have reports that contain local data | ■ Surveys of clients<br>■ Focus group with clients<br>■ Community forum events<br>■ Interviews with community leaders<br>■ Interviews with representatives of other health and social service agencies |

| *Type of Data* | *Examples of Existing Sources Outside Your Agency* | *Sources That Can Be Generated by Your Agency* |
|---|---|---|
| The relationship between specific skills, attitudes, and beliefs and HIV risk behavior | ■ CDC<br>*Compendium of HIV Prevention Interventions with Evidence of Effectiveness*<br>http://www.cdc.gov/hiv/pubs/hivcompendium/hivcompendium.htm<br>■ National Campaign to Prevent Teen Pregnancy publications<br>http://www.teenpregnancy.org<br>■ Journal articles; e.g., see:<br>National Library of Medicine<br>*PubMed Database*<br>http://www.ncbi.nlm.nih.gov/entrez/query.fcgi<br>■ Local universities, foundations, and public or private health and social service agencies may have reports that contain local data | ■ Surveys of clients<br>■ Focus group with clients<br>■ Community forum events<br>■ Interviews with community leaders<br>■ Interviews with representatives of other health and social service agencies |
| Local community norms and values | ■ Journal articles; e.g., see:<br>National Library of Medicine<br>*PubMed Database*<br>http://www.ncbi.nlm.nih.gov/entrez/query.fcgi<br>■ Local universities, foundations, and public or private health and social service agencies may have reports that contain local data | ■ Surveys of clients<br>■ Focus group with clients<br>■ Community forum events<br>■ Interviews with community leaders |
| Local laws, regulations, and policies | ■ State or local Public Health Department, Social Services Agency, or Department of Education publications or Web sites | ■ Interviews with representatives of other health and social service agencies |
| Current local prevention services | ■ Directories produced by local Public Health Departments or non-profit service agencies | ■ Interviews with representatives of other health and social service agencies |
| Effective prevention programs | ■ CDC<br>*Compendium of HIV Prevention Interventions with Evidence of Effectiveness*<br>http://www.cdc.gov/hiv/pubs/hivcompendium/hivcompendium.htm<br>■ CDC<br>*Replicating Effective Programs (REP)Plus*<br>http://www.cdc.gov/hiv/projects/rep/<br>■ CDC and the Academy for Educational Development (AED)<br>*Diffusion of Effective Behavioral Interventions (DEBI)*<br>http://www.effectiveinterventions.org/<br>■ Sociometrics Corporation<br>*HIV/AIDS Prevention Programs Archive (HAPPA)*<br>http://www.socio.com/happa.htm<br>■ Sociometrics Corporation<br>*Program Archive on Sexuality, Health and Adolescence (PASHA)*<br>http://www.socio.com/pasha.htm<br>■ National Campaign to Prevent Teen Pregnancy<br>http://www.teenpregnancy.org<br>■ Advocates for Youth<br>http://www.advocatesforyouth.org<br>■ Urban Institute<br>http://www.urban.org | ■ Review of evaluation data on your current HIV prevention programming |

| Type of Data | Examples of Existing Sources Outside Your Agency | Sources That Can Be Generated by Your Agency |
|---|---|---|
| Effective prevention programs (continued) | ■ ETR's ReCAPP Web site http://www.etr.org/recapp/ <br> ■ Reports by local public health departments on local programs that have been evaluated | |
| Funding opportunities | ■ Federal funding opportunities http://www.grants.gov/ <br> ■ The Foundation Center http://fdncenter.org/funders/ <br> ■ Web sites of private foundations | ■ Review of agency records to identify past funders or funder contacts |
| Other sources of program assistance (e.g., partners, volunteers, etc.) | ■ Web sites of local health, social service, and religious agencies and networks; Schools of Public Health at local universities; and private companies' corporate giving and volunteer programs | ■ Survey of community members to obtain feedback on interest in volunteering, donating equipment, etc. |

## Tool 2-5 Needs and Assets Data Collection and Analysis Planning Matrix[1]

It is important to plan your needs and assets assessment carefully. The matrix below will help you to do this.

To type directly into the matrix below on your computer (using the file on the CD-ROM), click on the gray-shaded area in the box you would like to type in. (Note that the gray shading will not appear in printouts of this document.) The boxes will expand as needed as you type. Alternately, you may photocopy this tool (for your use only) and complete it by hand or typewriter.

| Questions To Be Answered *(See Tool 2-3)* | Data to Obtain | Data Sources & Collection Methods *(See Tools 2-4 and 4-1)* | Who Will Collect the Data | Data Analysis Methods (Quantitative, Qualitative) | Who Will Analyze the Data | Timeframe |
|---|---|---|---|---|---|---|
| 1. | | | | | | |
| 2. | | | | | | |
| 3. | | | | | | |
| 4. | | | | | | |
| 5. | | | | | | |
| 6. | | | | | | |
| 7. | | | | | | |
| 8. | | | | | | |
| 9. | | | | | | |
| 10. | | | | | | |

[1] Adapted from Card, J. J., Brindis, C., Peterson, J. L., & Niego, S. (2001). *Guidebook: Evaluating teen pregnancy prevention programs* (2nd ed., Exercise 4.4). Los Altos, CA: Sociometrics Corporation.

## Tool 2-6 Matrix for Disseminating Needs and Assets Assessment Findings[1]

It is important to think through how you will disseminate the findings of your needs and assets assessment to key audiences. The matrix below will help you do this.

   To fill in the matrix on your computer (using the file on the CD-ROM), click on the gray-shaded area in the box you would like to type in. (Note that the gray shading will not appear in printouts of this document.) Alternately, you may photocopy this tool (for your use only) and complete it by hand or typewriter.

| Audience | Methods for Sharing Results, e.g.: <br> ■ *Report*  ■ *Newspaper article* <br> ■ *Report summary*  ■ *Agency Web site* <br> ■ *Fact sheet*  ■ *Meeting or event presentation* <br> ■ *Newsletter article*  ■ *Radio interview* | Who Will Take the Lead | Timeframe |
|---|---|---|---|
| **Colleagues at Your Agency** | | | |
| **Board of Directors** | | | |
| **Colleagues at Other Agencies** | | | |
| **Clients** | | | |
| **Other Community Members** | | | |
| **Community Leaders** | | | |
| **Policy Makers** | | | |
| **Funders** | | | |
| **Other** *(specify:)* | | | |

[1] Adapted from Card, J. J., Brindis, C., Peterson, J. L., & Niego, S. (2001). *Guidebook: Evaluating teen pregnancy prevention programs* (2nd ed., Exercise 4.5). Los Altos, CA: Sociometrics Corporation.

# Tool 2-7 Matrix for Involving Community Leaders in Program Planning[1]

It is important to think through how you will involve community leaders (e.g., community organizers or activists, religious leaders, community elders, neighborhood committee members, and others who are respected in the community) in your program planning efforts. The matrix below will help you do this.

To type directly into the matrix below (using the file on the CD-ROM), click on the gray-shaded area in the box you would like to type in. (Note that the gray shading will not appear in printouts of this document.) Alternately, you may photocopy this tool (for you use only) and complete it by hand or typewriter.

| Name of Community Leader | Contact Information | Areas of Interest or Expertise | Possible Program Planning Tasks, e.g.: ■ Needs assessment focus group member ■ Member of planning committee ■ Advocate for program in community |
|---|---|---|---|
|  |  |  |  |
|  |  |  |  |
|  |  |  |  |
|  |  |  |  |
|  |  |  |  |
|  |  |  |  |
|  |  |  |  |

---

[1] Adapted from Card, J. J., Brindis, C., Peterson, J. L., & Niego, S. (2001). *Guidebook: Evaluating teen pregnancy prevention programs* (2nd ed., Exercise 4.1). Los Altos, CA: Sociometrics Corporation.

## Tool 2-8 Problem Statement Development Worksheet

It is helpful to develop a brief problem statement that offers a succinct summary of the issues, problems, and needs facing a community. The problem statement provides the perspective needed for subsequent program planning activities.

To type directly into the boxes below (using the file on the CD-ROM), click on the gray-shaded area in the box you would like to type in. (Note that the gray shading will not appear in printouts of this document.) The boxes will expand as needed as you type. Alternately, you may photocopy this tool (for your use only) and complete it by hand or typewriter.

1. **What is your vision for your community? (Describe your vision or values stance.)**
(*Example:* "Our vision is that all people in our community will make healthy sexual decisions and avoid infection with HIV.")

2. **What is the affected population that you seek to address? (Describe your target population.)**
(*Example:* "In Newburgh City, young African-American women ages 19–29 have the highest rate of AIDS diagnosis across all cultural groups.")

3. **How significant is the problem? What are the consequences for community members? (Provide evidence for the scope of the problem.)**
(*Example:* "Over 50% of AIDS cases among Newburgh City residents occur among African-Americans under age 40. One out of 80 African-American females ages 19–29 is HIV+.")

4. **What causes the problem? (Indicate what key precursors are contributing to the problem, and what the gaps are between available and needed services.)**
(*Example:* "Due in part to gender-based socialization, young African-American women in our community lack the skills, self-efficacy, and motivation to negotiate safer sex successfully. Few programs offer a safe environment in which to address the factors contributing to HIV infection.")

5. **How should the problem be addressed? (Summarize potential solutions to the problem, based on scientific research and community perspectives. Include reference to solutions that you will seek to implement.)**
(*Example:* "Young women need opportunities to build skills, self-efficacy and motivation to engage in safer sex practices in ways that are culturally appropriate. Focus groups and the HIV prevention literature suggest that peer educator-led workshops [led by well-trained facilitators] can address this need.")

6. **How will we know the problem has been solved? (List one or two key indicators that will provide evidence of program success.)**
(*Example:* "We would expect program participants to increase safer sex practices, such as condom-protected sex, which will ultimately contribute to lower HIV infection rates in our community.")

7. **Using your responses to items 1–6, develop a succinct, two- to three-paragraph problem statement that summarizes the issue to be addressed in the community.**

## Tool 2-9 Goals and Objectives Planning Worksheet

This worksheet will help you to identify your program goals and objectives—what you want to change in the clients that you serve. After defining your target population(s), work from **right to left** to identify goals and objectives. If you have more than one target population (e.g., youth and their parents), be sure to specify goals and objectives for each. For each target population, draw arrows to show the links between the objectives and the goals you have identified.

   To type directly into the boxes below (using the file of the CD-ROM), click on the gray-shaded area in the box you would like to type in. (Note that the gray shading will not appear in printouts of this document.) The boxes will expand as needed as you type. Alternately, you may photocopy this tool (for your use only) and complete it by hand or typewriter.

| **Target population(s):** *Defined in terms of number, age, gender, ethnicity, etc.* | | |
|---|---|---|
| **Short-Term Objectives:** *Changes in knowledge, attitudes, skills, intentions, and behaviors that are potentially measurable on program completion or shortly thereafter.* | **Mid-Term Objectives:** *Changes in behaviors that are potentially measurable beginning several months to a year after program completion.* | **Long-Term Goals:** *Changes in behaviors or health status (e.g., STI/HIV infection) that are potentially measurable beginning a year or more after program completion.* |
| | | |

# Tool 2-10 Program Components Planning Worksheet

The matrix below will help you describe the activities or services that you will offer to your target population. An example is provided in first row.

To type directly into the boxes below (using the file on the CD-ROM), click on the gray-shaded area in the box you would like to type in. (Note that the gray shading will not appear in printouts of this document.) The boxes will expand as needed as you type. Alternately, you may photocopy this tool (for your use only) and complete it by hand or typewriter.

| Component | Approach | Content | Delivery methods | Duration and frequency | Setting | Staffing |
|---|---|---|---|---|---|---|
| HIV prevention workshop series | HIV education & behavioral skills-building | Session 1. What HIV and AIDS are; how HIV is transmitted; and how it can be prevented; what HIV testing involves; how AIDS is treated Session 2. Safer sex communication, negotiation, and refusal skills; condom use skills Session 3. Coping skills: how to engage in safer sex while coping with partner rejection and effects of alcohol and drug use; provision of support resource information | Each session includes: presentation, role playing, group discussion, video | Once a week for 2 hours over a 3-week period The workshop cycle is offered six times per year | A meeting room at our agency | Two health educators, one male and one female, each devoting 20% of his/her time to the program |
| | | | | | | |
| | | | | | | |
| | | | | | | |
| | | | | | | |
| | | | | | | |

## Tool 2-11 Program Model Development Worksheet

This worksheet will help you to **put your program model together** (Part I) and **assess its strength** (Part II).

## Part I. Develop the Model

After describing your target population(s) below, remember to work from *right to left* to fill in your goals and objectives (per Tool 2–9) and your program components (per Tool 2–10).

To type directly into the boxes below (using the file on the CD-ROM), click on the gray-shaded area in the box you would like to type in. (Note that the gray shading will not appear in printouts of this document.) The boxes will expand as needed as you type. You may then wish to print the model so that you can draw in arrows to show the links among components, objectives, and goals. Alternately, you may photocopy this tool (for your use only) and complete it by hand or typewriter.

| **Target population(s):** *Defined in terms of number, age, gender, ethnicity, etc.* | | | |
| --- | --- | --- | --- |
| **Program Components:** *Activities or services to be provided (summary of content, delivery methods, duration, etc.)* | **Short-Term Objectives:** *Immediate changes in knowledge, attitudes, skills, intentions, and behaviors.* | **Mid-Term Objectives:** *Mid-term changes in behaviors.* | **Long-Term Goals:** *Long-term changes in behaviors or health status (e.g., STI/HIV infection).* |
| | | | |

## Part II. Assess Model Strength

To assess model strength, discuss the questions below with your key stakeholders. You may wish to make notes on the discussion as you go and then place an "x" in each checkbox (□) as you complete discussion of that question. To place an "x" in the checkboxes on your computer (using the file on your CD-ROM), use your cursor to click on the box. To remove an "x" from a box, click on the box again.

□ **To what extent does the model address HIV-related needs and assets of the target population, local community, and agency?**
*Notes:*

□ **How robustly are cultural factors influencing HIV risk addressed?**
*Notes:*

□ **Is the intervention consistent with local cultural norms?**
*Notes:*

□ **Does the model present a coherent theory of change?**
*Notes:*

□ **How strong are the links among program components, objectives, and goals?**
*Notes:*

□ **How robustly does the model incorporate characteristics common to effective programs?**
*Notes:*

□ **Is there consensus on the model among key stakeholders?**
*Notes:*

# Tool 2-12 Replication Decision-Making Worksheet

This worksheet will help you to decide *whether* to replicate an HIV prevention program that was developed elsewhere, as well as *which* program to replicate.

 To type directly into the boxes below (using the file on the CD-ROM), click on the gray-shaded area in the box you would like to type in. (Note that the gray shading will not appear in printouts of this document.) The boxes will expand as needed as you type. Alternately, you may photocopy this tool (for your use only) and complete it by hand or typewriter.

## PART I. COLLECT INFORMATION ABOUT CANDIDATE PROGRAMS

| CRITERION: | YOUR ASSESSMENT OF PROGRAM #1: | YOUR ASSESSMENT OF PROGRAM #2: | YOUR ASSESSMENT OF PROGRAM #3: |
|---|---|---|---|
| **1. Appropriateness of health status goals** *Appropriateness of candidate programs' long-term health status goals (e.g., to reduce STIs) for your target population, community, and agency context* | | | |
| **2. Appropriateness of behavioral objectives** *Appropriateness of candidate programs' short- and mid-term behavioral objectives (e.g., to increase consistent condom use) for your target population, community, and agency context* | | | |
| **3. Appropriateness of nonbehavioral objectives** *Appropriateness of candidate programs' nonbehavioral objectives (i.e., desired changes in knowledge, attitudes, intentions, and skills) for your target population, community, and agency context* | | | |
| **4. Appropriateness of activities or services** *Appropriateness of candidate programs' activities or services for your target population* | | | |
| **5. Appropriateness of program materials** *Appropriateness of candidate programs' workbooks, videos, and other materials for your target population* | | | |
| **6. Similarity of original to new target population** *Similarity of candidate programs' target population to your target population, especially with respect to:* ■ *developmental level* ■ *HIV risk level* ■ *cultural factors influencing HIV risk* | | | |
| **7. Strength of evaluation evidence** *Strength of evidence of candidate programs' effectiveness in achieving their objectives and goals, especially with a population similar to your target population* | | | |

| CRITERION: | YOUR ASSESSMENT OF PROGRAM #1: | YOUR ASSESSMENT OF PROGRAM #2: | YOUR ASSESSMENT OF PROGRAM #3: |
|---|---|---|---|
| **8. Incorporation of characteristics of effective programs** *Candidate programs' degree of incorporation of characteristics common to effective programs that have taken the same approach (e.g., HIV education, counseling and testing, etc.)* | | | |
| **9. Agency philosophy and resources** *Appropriateness of candidate programs for agency philosophy and resources, including:* • *staffing (number, credentials)* • *funding* • *time with target population* • *facilities* | | | |
| **10. Availability of program materials** *Availability of candidate programs' materials* | *Indicate whether/how materials can be acquired:* | *Indicate whether/how materials can be acquired:* | *Indicate whether/how materials can be acquired:* |

## PART II. ASSESS FEASIBILITY OF REPLICATING CANDIDATE PROGRAMS

Answer the following questions based on the information you collected in Part I. To place an "x" in the square box (☐) next to your answer selections on your computer (using the file on the CD-ROM), use your cursor to click on the box. To remove an "x" from a box, click on the box again.

| NAMES OF CANDIDATE PROGRAMS → | #1: | #2: | #3: |
|---|---|---|---|
| 1. How good is the overall fit of each candidate program for your target population, community context, and agency? | ☐ excellent<br>☐ good<br>☐ fair<br>☐ poor | ☐ excellent<br>☐ good<br>☐ fair<br>☐ poor | ☐ excellent<br>☐ good<br>☐ fair<br>☐ poor |
| 2. Would replicating the candidate program require you to make fundamental changes to program objectives and components or more surface-level changes to materials? | ☐ fundamental changes<br>☐ surface changes | ☐ fundamental changes<br>☐ surface changes | ☐ fundamental changes<br>☐ surface changes |
| 3. Would you have the resources to make program adaptations to reduce mismatches between the program and your target population, community context, and agency? *(See also Tool 2–13: Adaptation Checklist.)* | ☐ yes<br>☐ maybe<br>☐ no | ☐ yes<br>☐ maybe<br>☐ no | ☐ yes<br>☐ maybe<br>☐ no |
| 4a. Would the original developer or evaluator of the program be available to provide assistance with adaptation?<br>b. If so, how much time could s/he devote, and how much would it cost your agency? | ☐ yes- if so, indicate:<br>time:<br>cost:<br>☐ no | ☐ yes- if so, indicate:<br>time:<br>cost:<br>☐ no | ☐ yes- if so, indicate:<br>time:<br>cost:<br>☐ no |
| 5. Do your funders favor replication of an existing program or development of a new or hybrid program? | ☐ Favor replication<br>☐ Favor new/hybrid program<br>☐ No preference | ☐ Favor replication<br>☐ Favor new/hybrid program<br>☐ No preference | ☐ Favor replication<br>☐ Favor new/hybrid program<br>☐ No preference |

**Based on your answers, which (if any) of the candidate programs would be most suitable for replication by your agency?**

> *Fill in name of program(s):*

## PART III. ADDRESS REPLICATION CHALLENGES

**If you have decided to replicate a program, what challenges do you expect to face? What are some strategies you might use to address these challenges?**

| Challenges | Strategies |
|---|---|
| 1. | |
| 2. | |
| 3. | |
| 4. | |
| 5. | |

# Tool 2-13 Adaptation Checklist

Adapting an effective program (i.e., one that has shown positive behavioral or health status effects through rigorous outcome evaluation) to meet the needs of your target population and setting can be a good programming strategy. When undertaking adaptation of an effective program, it is important to reduce mismatches between the original program and the new context without undermining the core program, or those elements that are responsible for the program's effectiveness. This checklist will help you to adapt an effective program in a systematic and culturally competent way.

Place an "x" in the square box (□) as you complete each item. (To do this on your computer—using the file in your CD-ROM—use your cursor to click on the box. To remove an "x" from a box, click on the box again.)

□ **1. Assemble an adaptation planning team that includes program staff and representatives of your target population or local community.**

□ **2. Develop (or obtain from the program developer) a program model for the original program that identifies:**
- Program goals and objectives (i.e., desired changes in the target population).
- Program components (i.e., activities or services).
- Links among the goals, objectives, and program components.
  *(Note: see also Tool 2-11: Program Model Development Worksheet.)*

□ **3. Identify the core program.**
   □ Are there any *research studies* (documented in evaluation reports or journal articles) that have demonstrated what elements of the program are essential to its success?
   □ Based on the *formal theory* that underlies the program, what behavioral and non-behavioral goals/objectives and program components are essential to program success?
   □ Based on the *experiences of the original program developer/evaluator*, what elements of the program are essential to program success?

□ **4. Mark core program elements on the program model.**

□ **5. Review each column of the program model from right to left. As you do so, make adaptations to the elements of the model to reduce mismatches with your context. Some potential sources of mismatch may include:**
   □ Characteristics of clients
      □ Developmental level
      □ Level of behavioral risk
      □ Cultural norms and values
      □ Language background
      □ Literacy level
   □ Characteristics of agencies
      □ Philosophy
      □ Staff credentials/expertise
      □ Staff cultural competence
      □ Available resources (e.g., funding, facilities, time with target population)
   □ Characteristics of communities
      □ Cultural norms and values
      □ Laws, regulations, or policies (e.g., concerning needle exchange)
      □ Infrastructure (e.g., transportation)

□ **6. Assess the revised model according to each of the following:**
   □ Does the model present a coherent theory of change?
   □ How strong are the links among program components, objectives, and goals?
   □ Does the model retain fidelity to core components?
   □ Does the model robustly incorporate characteristics common to effective programs that have taken similar approaches or been used successfully with similar populations?
   □ Does the model address HIV-related needs and assets of the target population, local community, and agency?

☐ How robustly are cultural factors affecting HIV risk addressed?
☐ Is the intervention consistent with local cultural norms?
☐ Is there consensus on the model among the planning team?

☐ **7. Revise program materials in accordance with the adapted model.**
☐ Materials should reflect the revised program components.
☐ Materials should be appropriate for participants':
☐ Developmental level
☐ Level of behavioral risk
☐ Cultural norms and values
☐ Language background
☐ Literacy level *(Note: See also Tool 3–4: Checklist for Developing Effective Print Materials for Low-Literacy Populations)*

☐ **8. Plan for staffing issues that are specific to your context.**
☐ Recruit staff with appropriate experience and skills.
☐ Train staff in:
☐ Content of the adapted program
☐ Delivery format of the adapted program
☐ Cultural competence

☐ **9. Plan for participant recruitment issues that are specific to your context.**
*(Note: See also Tool 3–2: Participant Recruitment Checklist)*

# Tool 2-14 Template for Preparing a Position Announcement

This worksheet will help you to prepare an announcement for a program staff position.

To fill in the table below on your computer (using the file on the CD-ROM), click on the gray-shaded area in the box you would like to type in. (Note that the gray shading will not appear in printouts of this document.) The boxes will expand as needed as you type. Alternately, you may photocopy this tool (for your use only) and complete it by hand or typewriter.

| Announcement Section | Description |
| --- | --- |
| 1. **Agency, program, and client background** <br> *Brief background information on the history, mission, focus, location, and size of your agency, and your program's goals, activities, and clients.* | |
| 2. **Position duties** <br> *A summary of position responsibilities, start date, and indication of whether the position is:* <br> ■ *For an employee, consultant, or volunteer.* <br> ■ *Temporary or long-term.* <br> ■ *Part-time or full-time.* | |
| 3. **Key qualifications** <br> *Information on the educational or professional credentials, skills, experience, and other qualities that are required or preferred.* | |
| 4. **Compensation** <br> *Summary information on salary (or salary range) and benefits.* | |
| 5. **Application procedures and deadlines** <br> ■ *List of materials to be submitted.* <br> ■ *Instructions on how, by when, and to whom to submit them.* <br> ■ *Timeline for notification of candidates (if known).* | |

# Tool 2-15 Template for Assessing Candidates

This template will help you to think about criteria for assessing the candidates for a program staff position.

To fill in the table below on your computer (using the file on the CD-ROM), click on the gray-shaded area in the box you would like to type in. (Note that the gray shading will not appear in printouts of this document.) The boxes will expand as needed as you type. Alternately, you may photocopy this tool (for your use only) and complete it by hand or typewriter.

| | |
|---|---|
| **Program staff position:** | |
| **Name of candidate:** | |

| Criterion | Position Requirements and Preferences | Candidate's Information |
|---|---|---|
| **Educational or professional credentials** *(e.g., BA degree, CHES certification)* | | |
| **Prior experience** *(Length and nature of responsibilities, including involvement with specific populations)* | | |
| **Additional skills** *(e.g., Language background, software use, etc.)* | | |
| **Feedback from candidate's references** | *[NA]* | |
| **Other** *(Specify:)* | | |

| |
|---|
| **Summary of candidate's match for position:** |

# Culturally Competent Program Implementation

## OVERVIEW

*Culturally competent program implementation* involves community leaders in program activities, monitors ongoing and emerging target population needs, makes appropriate mid-course program adjustments to meet these needs, addresses barriers to effective communication among participants and staff, encourages participant and staff feedback, and respects the cultural norms and diversity of staff, clients, and community members. This section will cover the following six topics:

## 1. Involving Community Leaders in Implementation

A culturally competent HIV prevention program utilizes the talents and skills of local community members in its implementation. Involving key community leaders in recruiting and retaining participants, serving as volunteer program educators, organizing community education events, and monitoring and refining program activities to meet target population needs are some ways to enhance the cultural competence of your program implementation.

## 2. Recruiting and Retaining Program Participants

Developing and implementing focused recruitment and retention strategies for your target population can help improve program attendance and completion rates. Useful recruitment methods include posting ads at sites frequented by your target population, or in local newspapers, magazines, or online listservs; making presentations at community events; sending outreach workers to target population "hang-outs"; cross-marketing with other agencies; and providing age- and culturally appropriate enrollment incentives. Helpful retention strategies include providing tangible rewards for program attendance; incorporating fun and appropriate social activities; and making appropriate mid-course adjustments to address client needs.

## 3. Responding to Target Population Needs

Barriers that affect program participation range from such *logistical factors* as inaccessible program times or locations, high program fees, and lack of bilingual staff to such *perceived factors* as discomfort with program topics or staff and concerns about confidentiality. Monitoring ongoing clients needs by reviewing attendance data and soliciting participant and staff feedback can help generate ideas about how to address these needs. It is important to use this information to make mid-course program adjustments so that the program delivery is improved in a timely fashion.

## 4. Addressing Language Barriers

Language barriers can present a significant challenge to HIV prevention service agencies that work with culturally diverse populations. Language barriers can affect program access, client-provider communication, and health outcomes. Means to address these barriers include hiring more bilingual/bicultural staff; engaging professional interpreters; and translating program materials into primary participant language(s). It is also important to attend to related culturally based communication norms, such as body language and respectful forms of address. When target populations have low literacy levels, developing print materials with abundant visual aids can help.

## 5. Retaining Program Staff

Staff retention is an important challenge for HIV prevention programs. Attention to staff-management communication, staff training, ongoing staff support and feedback, and staff recognition and rewards can decrease staff turnover rates. Specific strategies include periodic, in-person individual meetings with staff; providing ongoing training on relevant topics; regularly soliciting and acting on staff input; and hosting events that show appreciation for staff.

## 6. Practicing Culturally Competent Program Management

Managing an HIV prevention program involves many tasks: promoting culturally competent programming, overseeing day-to-day operations, ensuring adequate staffing, tracking resource use, reporting on program delivery and outcomes, writing grant proposals, and often simultaneously serving as a direct service provider. Because program managers are in positions of influence, it is important that they set an example for how to interact effectively with clients and community members and work to create a culturally competent program environment.

## INVOLVING COMMUNITY LEADERS IN IMPLEMENTATION

### Why Involving Community Leaders in Program Implementation Is Important

As was described in Section 2, a *community leader* is anyone whom group members identify as their representative or someone they respect, such as an elected leader, community organizer or activist, religious leader, elder, or peer group opinion leader. As people who are respected and looked up to, community leaders have the important ability to mobilize group members to support or participate in programs, campaigns, or processes. They can also provide helpful input on how to refine ongoing programs so that they are maximally appropriate for and appealing to their target audiences.

### Identifying Community Leaders

As was discussed in Section 2, community leaders can be identified in a variety of ways, such as through program staff's contacts in the community, contacts at other service agencies and community-based organizations, focus groups with current or former clients, participation in community events or activities, and outreach activities at local community sites.

It is important to remember that because members of any community have diverse cultural and social affiliations, not everyone in a given community will agree on who their leaders are (Butterfoss et al., 1996). You need to be sure that you identify leaders within the various *subgroups* of your target community (e.g., Spanish-only speakers, bilingual individuals, and English-only speakers, if you are working with diverse Latino populations). This will help ensure that your program is reaching and meeting the needs of all members of your target population.

## Community Leaders as Resources for Program Implementation

There are many possible ways to involve community leaders in program implementation efforts, for example:

- As outreach workers for client recruitment and retention activities.
- As lay health educators.
- As organizers of—or speakers at—program-related community events.
- As advocates who generate community support for the program.
- As members of a team that monitors and refines program activities to better address participant needs.

For some roles, such as that of peer educator or outreach worker, it may be necessary to train community leaders in activity content and delivery methods before they begin to conduct their program work. Such training has the added benefit of helping community leaders to acquire new skills (e.g., presentation or facilitation skills) that may be of use to them in other areas of their lives. Tool 3–1: Matrix for Involving Community Leaders in Program Implementation can facilitate your identification and involvement of community leaders in program implementation.

In addition to serving as valuable resources for HIV prevention program implementation, community leaders can also benefit from participation in program implementation efforts. For example, a study of gay Latinos' volunteer involvement in HIV/AIDS-related organizations in Chicago found that volunteers reported increased self-esteem, sense of empowerment, and safer sex behaviors (Ramirez-Valles & Brown, 2003). Through their program involvement, community leaders may also sharpen their presentation and leadership skills, expand their networks, and gather knowledge and experience that they can apply to other projects. Promoting these benefits, and ensuring that community leaders participate in stimulating, personally meaningful activities, can help to improve recruitment and retention of such leaders in program implementation efforts.

## RECRUITING AND RETAINING PROGRAM PARTICIPANTS

Recruiting and retaining participants are critical activities for any HIV prevention program effort. After all, you cannot conduct an intervention without participants, and resources are wasted if services are not reaching the desired population.

Participant recruitment and retention can, however, be challenging. It is a good idea to develop and implement specific, focused recruitment and retention strategies that address the norms and circumstances of your target population.

## Recruitment

*Recruitment* refers to locating, earning the trust of, and enrolling members of your target audience in your HIV prevention program. Successful recruitment depends in part on planning a program that appropriately addresses target population preferences and needs with respect to timing, location, content, delivery methods, and staffing. But successful recruitment also depends on your ability to publicize the program in culturally appropriate and appealing ways.

There are a number of methods you can consider when developing a recruitment strategy. These include (Conner et al., 2005; Janz et al., 1996; Lehman, 2002; Wakefield, 2001):

- Producing **recruitment materials and outreach protocols in all the primary languages** of your target population. These materials should include culturally appropriate messages and images.
- Posting fliers with information about your program at **sites frequented by your target population**. For example, if you are working with youth, such sites might include schools, parks, youth centers, arcades, or other popular after-school hang-outs.
- Making **presentations** or hosting **information booths** at local community events, such as festivals, street fairs, and Parent Teacher Association (PTA) meetings.
- Sending **outreach workers** to populations exhibiting high-risk behaviors.
- Working with other community agencies to **cross-market** your program to their clients.
- Posting **ads** in local newspapers, magazines, or e-mail listservs that are popular among your target population.
- Holding an **"open house" event** that affords community members the opportunity to meet your staff and learn about your services in an informal context.
- Offering a **toll-free telephone number and Web site** for easy initial contact with the program.
- Providing age- and culturally appropriate **incentives** for program enrollment, such as T-shirts, caps, key chains, or phone cards printed with your program logo.
- Providing services such as **transportation** (or transportation vouchers) and **child care** (for participants with young children) to reduce potential barriers to participation.

Community leaders can help you to identify and implement specific recruitment methods that will be effective with your population. Tool 3–2: Participant Recruitment Checklist can help you keep track of the methods you select and what needs to be done to implement each.

## Retention

*Program retention* refers to the extent to which programs are able to retain their participants until the end of a program cycle or during a given period of time. Participant retention is vital to program success but is often more challenging than participant recruitment. Those who initially attend a program may later drop out because of competing activities and priorities (e.g., work, child care responsibilities, after-school activities, etc.); cognitive challenges (e.g., because of substance use or mental health problems); or transportation difficulties. They may also fail to complete the program due to a sense of boredom, disconnect, discomfort, or dissatisfaction with program staff, content, or delivery methods.

As in the case of program recruitment, high retention rates are in part dependent on your having planned a program that addresses your target population's preferences and needs. However, a number of actions designed specifically to promote program retention can help ensure that clients who initially attend the program come back for subsequent sessions. Examples of retention strategies include (Brown-Peterside et al., 2001; Harris et al., 2003; Villarruel et al., 2006):

- **Providing transportation.** Provide bus passes, subway tokens, van service, or other resources to help clients get to the service location.
- **Making child care available.** For participants with young children, having free, reliable child care available onsite can make the difference between sticking with the program and dropping out.
- **Offering incentives.** Reward attendance with items such as food, gift cards, or T-shirts. Provide a graduation certificate and ceremony for those who complete the program to recognize their accomplishment.
- **Making referrals to other services.** Provide counseling or referrals to clients who are facing multiple challenges, such substance use, mental illness, homelessness, unemployment, or domestic violence or other abuse. This can help build trust and ultimately reduce a range of barriers that keep clients from participating fully in HIV prevention services.
- **Planning appropriate social activities**. Offer culturally appropriate parties, holiday celebrations, and other activities that build a sense of trust, social support, and engagement with others. This can help create a sense of community that makes program attendance more appealing.
- **Making personalized contact.** Consider calling, sending e-mail, writing a letter, or visiting clients where they live or spend time if they miss sessions or stop attending the program. Ask why they have not been participating in the program and take whatever steps you can to address their concerns or needs so that they are able to return. (However, be sure not to put clients' confidentiality or personal safety at risk by making others aware of their participation in HIV/AIDS-related services.)

Some of these strategies are also helpful for participant recruitment, as was indicated earlier. As in the case of participant recruitment, community leaders can help you to decide what program retention activities would be most effective with your target population.

Tale 3–1 provides an example of how a variety of factors can support or hinder participation of Latino youth in an HIV prevention intervention, and what can be done to address these factors. Tool 3–3: Participant Retention Checklist can help you keep track of the retention methods you select and what needs to be done to implement each.

## RESPONDING TO TARGET POPULATION NEEDS

### Factors That Affect Program Implementation

With careful planning, it is possible to anticipate many needs and preferences of your target population. For example, you can schedule program activities at times when clients are most likely to be available and willing to attend. You can also acquire or develop materials in clients' native languages, and include culturally appropriate visuals. However, even the most detail-oriented program planners will seldom be able to anticipate and address all of the potential barriers that may affect program participation. As was mentioned in Section 2, these can include both logistical and perceived barriers (Brindis & Davis, 1998). Logistical barriers are physical impediments, such as inaccessible program locations and times, fees that clients cannot afford; and shortage of staff who are fluent in the range of client languages. Perceived barriers, in contrast, are psychological impediments, such as the belief that the program is not relevant or interesting, discomfort with program staff due to different cultural backgrounds, concern about confidentiality of personal

## 3-1    Recruitment and Retention of Latino Youth for the ¡Cuídate! Program

Antonia Villarruel and her colleagues from the University of Michigan and the University of Pennsylvania recognized the need for culturally tailored HIV prevention interventions for Latino adolescents. With extensive input from Latino parents, teens, community leaders, and service providers in Detroit and Philadelphia, they adapted the *Be Proud! Be Responsible!* curriculum, which had been shown to be effective with inner-city African-American adolescents (Jemmott et al., 1992; Jemmott et al., 1995). The new program, called *¡Cuídate! Latin Youth Health Promotion Program, was developed in both English- and Spanish-language versions* for use with inner-city Latinos ages 13–18. The team then set out to design culturally appropriate participant recruitment and retention strategies that would support successful implementation and evaluation of the program.

Like the *Be Proud! Be Responsible! Program, ¡Cuídate! is based on social cognitive theory* and the theories of reasoned action and planned behavior (see Chapter 2). Additionally, both programs include six modules designed to influence knowledge, attitudes, beliefs, skills, behaviors, and self-efficacy with regard to HIV risk reduction (including negotiation of abstinence and condom use). However, unlike *Be Proud! Be Responsible!, ¡Cuídate!* incorporates key aspects of Latino culture by discussing how cultural concepts such as *familialism* (the importance of family) and gender roles influence HIV risk. Cultural values that support safer sex are highlighted, and those that are perceived as barriers to safer sex are reframed. For example, although *machismo* is stereotypically associated with a man doing whatever he wants and making decisions for others, in the curriculum it is presented as placing value on protecting others and keeping the family safe. The curriculum also presents information on HIV/AIDS risk and prevalence among Latinos (Villarruel et al., 2005).

Although the developers of *¡Cuídate!* realized the importance of culturally appropriate participant recruitment and retention strategies, they found few studies in the literature describing strategies specific to Latino teens. The team there-fore decided to develop and test their own tailored recruitment and retention approaches, in conjunction with an evaluation of the *¡Cuídate!* program. In doing so, the team worked closely with several high schools and community agencies in Philadelphia and with local Latino community leaders (Villarruel et al., 2006a).

Villarruel and colleagues took a number of steps to build a strong, culturally competent recruitment and retention approach for their study. In particular:

- They developed relationships with local Latino community leaders years prior to program implementation.
- They ensured that all program materials and related communication (e.g., registration slips, letters to parents and students, consent forms) were available in both English and Spanish.
- They recruited and hired program facilitators and project assistants from local Latino community-based agencies and schools.
- They hired bilingual/bicultural recruitment and retention specialists.
- To promote both recruitment and retention, they provided students with a program T-shirt and monetary compensation for participating in the intervention sessions and follow-up data collection activities.

High school personnel were especially helpful with recruitment. For example, they allowed the project's recruitment specialists to familiarize students with the program at assemblies and lunchtime. They also agreed to offer a community/service credit (which was necessary for graduation) to students who participated in the study.

Once recruited from local high schools and community-based organizations, interested participants were randomly assigned to either the *¡Cuídate!* program or to a general health promotion intervention control group. The programs were implemented on two consecutive Saturdays at participating high schools. Survey data on sexual activity and condom use were collected from all participants immediately before intervention participation, immediately after intervention participation, and at 3-, 6-, and 12-month follow-ups. Study retention strategies included:

- Asking participants to provide contact information at program registration, both for themselves and for a responsible adult who did not live with them but who would be able to contact them.
- Sending birthday and holiday cards with the program logo during the study.
- Sending reminder postcards and making reminder phone calls before each follow-up program and data collection session.
- Using consistent personnel to contact participants, so that they and their families could develop *confianza* (trust) and connection with a project team member.

Participant retention was high during the intervention period—the retention rate for the two HIV prevention sessions was 96% and the rate for the two health promotion intervention sessions was 94%. Retention at 3-month follow-up data collection was 82% and 86%, respectively, and retention at 12-month follow-up was 80% and 84%, respectively. Among participants lost to follow-up, many could not be contacted because they had dropped out of the school system, changed residences, had no forwarding address, and/or had provided invalid contact information.

To understand what other factors made it hard or easy for participants to attend follow-up sessions, the project team asked a random selection of 3-month follow-up participants to respond to several open-ended questions about study participation. Commonly cited *barriers* included:

- Jobs and responsibility for caring for children (e.g., younger siblings).
- Timing of follow-up or length of the follow-up questionnaire.
- Personal reasons, such as shyness about talking about sex and lack of friends in the group or lack of family support to participate.

Major *facilitators* to participation included:

- Positive peer pressure and family influences.
- Program incentives (money, school credit, and spending time with friends).
- Commitment to parents, friends, or school.
- The desire to help friends or younger siblings by passing information on to them.

Villarruel and her colleagues took away several lessons from the study that can be applied to future recruitment and retention efforts focused on Latino adolescents:

1. Culturally competent strategies for recruiting and retaining participants need to reflect the values of the target population and larger community. For example, retention was supported by the cultural value of familialism, reflected in the students' desire to share what they learned in the program with peers and siblings.
2. Recruitment and retention strategies should build *confianza* (trust) in the program and its staff and encourage ongoing community, school, and family involvement in and support for the program.
3. The program or study team must be able to communicate and incorporate values that are important to the target population and community—such as *respeto* (respect) for both the students and their families (Villarruel et al., 2006a).

It is also worth noting that the study's outcome evaluation yielded a number of very encouraging findings among participants. Over the 12-month follow-up period, *¡Cuídate!* participants were less likely to report sexual intercourse, multiple partners, and days of unprotected sex than control group participants. In addition, *¡Cuídate!* participants were more likely than control group participants to report using condoms consistently. Among Spanish-speakers, specifically, *¡Cuídate!* participants were also more likely to have used a condom at last sex and had a significantly higher proportion of protected sex acts than control group participants (Villarruel et al., 2006b). As such, *¡Cuídate!* is one of the first U.S.-based programs to demonstrate positive, long-term effects on Latino adolescents' sexual behavior.

information shared, and fear of arrest (e.g., for admitting drug use) or deportation (e.g., among undocumented persons).

It is important to bear in mind that environmental and cultural factors that affect program participation, service delivery quality, and client outcomes may change during program implementation (Castro et al., 2004; Kennedy et al., 2001; Sumartojo, 2000). Examples of these factors include:

- **Laws or policies**, such as minors' access to confidential reproductive and sexual health services, or the availability of syringes without a prescription.
- **Media coverage**, such as portrayals of HIV infection rates and risk levels, and portrayals of local HIV prevention and treatment service quality.
- **New fads**, such as the spread of new "club drugs" or popularity of new venues (such as the Internet) for meeting potential sexual partners.

Culturally competent program implementation takes steps to monitor such factors and to make mid-course program delivery changes that address client needs.

## Monitoring Client Needs

During your program, you can monitor ongoing or emerging client needs in a number of ways. For example, it is helpful to:

- **Record and review program registration and attendance data**. Checking periodically to see who is and who is not attending will indicate whether or not you are reaching your target population and can suggest whose needs are being met or unmet.
- **Obtain client feedback**. Feedback both from clients who attend the program regularly and those who attend sporadically or drop out can shed light on met and unmet needs as well. Focus groups, written surveys, and an anonymous "suggestion box" are common ways of obtaining such feedback. Be sure that you use methods that are culturally appropriate for your population.
- **Obtain staff feedback**. It is also useful to ask staff to note challenges to active client participation and effective program delivery. For example: Do some participants seem bored or disengaged? Do they raise questions or issues that are not addressed by the curriculum? Do communication difficulties arise due to different language backgrounds or interactional styles?

Collecting and analyzing these types of data are a part of process evaluation, which is discussed in further detail in Section 4.

## Addressing Client Needs

Once you have collected data on emerging clients' needs and issues, it is helpful to meet with staff and community leaders to prioritize the needs and issues, identify their root causes, brainstorm ways to address them, and agree on specific action steps. For example, let's say that your HIV prevention program involves three small group workshop sessions designed for men and women. However, during the just-completed first cycle of the program, only women attended. Table 3–1 shows some possible reasons for the lack of male participation, and a possible action step for each.

In practice, many programs wait until the end of a program or program cycle to address mismatches between service delivery and client needs. However, to bring

Possible Causes of—and Responses to—an HIV Prevention
Program Being Attended by Women Only

| Possible Cause | Possible Response |
|---|---|
| Recruitment efforts failed to reach males. | Post recruitment announcements in places frequented by men. |
| Males are unable to attend at the time the program is offered. | Consider changing the program time to better accommodate everyone's schedules. |
| Males are uninterested in the program or are not comfortable participating in the program with women. | Tailor the activity content and delivery formats for gender-specific groups, each with a gender-matched facilitator. |

the greatest benefit to your clients, it can be useful to consider what mid-course program changes might be made, within the bounds of available resources.

An example of how a program was adapted during implementation to better meet client needs is provided in Tale 3–2. Tool 3–4: Worksheet for Responding to Target Population Needs can help you respond to the issues that prevent your own program clients from deriving maximal benefit from your program.

## ADDRESSING LANGUAGE BARRIERS

### The Scope of Language Diversity in the United States

According to the 2000 U.S. Census (Shin & Bruno, 2003):

- 18% of the U.S. population (age 5 and over), or a total of 47 million people, speaks a language other than English at home.
- Of these 47 million people, 28 million speak Spanish at home. The remainder speak over 300 other languages.
- 4.4 million households, encompassing 11.9 million people, *are linguistically isolated*—that is, no household member age 14 or over self-identifies as speaking English "very well."

Language barriers present a significant resource challenge to HIV prevention service agencies that work with culturally diverse populations. For example, Asian and Pacific Islander (API) groups in the United States speak over 100 languages and dialects. Because 75% of APIs in the United States have little or no English proficiency, HIV prevention messages need to be made available in multiple languages to reach API communities effectively (The Body, 2004).

### Consequences of Language Barriers

Language barriers have significant implications for health care, including HIV prevention and treatment services (Bat-Chava et al., 2005; The Body, 2004; Grantmakers in Health, 2005; Santos et al., 2004; Scott et al., 2005). Specifically, language barriers have been shown to impede access to health insurance, preventive services, and treatment. Persons with limited English proficiency may be unaware of services or may avoid them because they expect communication problems with staff. Language barriers can also prevent clients from understanding oral or written prevention messages or treatment instructions. In addition, they can prevent clients from asking questions and providing feedback to service providers on their satisfaction with

## 3-2  Adapting the Popular Opinion Leaders (POL) Program During Implementation to Address Client Needs

Robin Miller and colleagues from New York City's Gay Men's Health Crisis (GMHC) were concerned about the high-risk behaviors taking place in hustler bars, local bars where male prostitutes meet their male clients. The research team decided that hustler bars would be a promising location for implementing an adapted version of the *Popular Opinion Leaders* (POL) program (Miller, 2003; see also Figure 2–12).

The original POL program was designed by Jeff Kelly and colleagues at the Medical College of Wisconsin to reduce unprotected sex among male patrons of gay bars. POL uses popular opinion leaders (i.e., bar patrons that other patrons look up to) to deliver safer sex messages, supporting the idea that safer sex is the norm among respected and admired people. Intervention delivery steps include: (1) training bartenders to identify natural leaders among patrons; (2) recruiting patrons who had been nominated by several bartenders as opinion leaders; (3) training the opinion leaders to deliver safer sex messages to their peers; and (4) making a contract with each opinion leader to have a specified number of conversations with his peers. The POL program has shown promising results in lowering rates of unprotected anal intercourse among bar patrons who have participated in the intervention (Kelly et al., 1991; Kelly et al., 1992; Kelly et al., 1997; see also Figure 3–1).

Overall, the POL program seemed well suited for the culture of hustler bars. However, the program planning team also realized some program adaptations were in order. First, training sessions needed to address situations that prostitutes might encounter, such as being offered more money for sex without a condom. Second, the training timeframe would have to accommodate hustlers' unusual and irregular schedules. Third, opinion leader activities (such as completion of evaluation paperwork) should be supported by providing trained volunteer liaisons who were familiar with the hustler community (Miller, 2003).

The program team knew they wanted to conduct the program with maximum fidelity (or faithfulness) to the original POL program and to their plans for the revised intervention. During program implementation, however, it became clear that some additional changes were needed to address the needs of opinion leaders and their clients. For example, in the program planning phase, the program team had recognized that opinion leaders' literacy levels tended to be low, so they tailored their training materials accordingly. In spite of these efforts, during program implementation, many opinion leaders were still unable to read all the materials and complete additional reading homework. This made it difficult for the opinion leaders to utilize the communication skills taught in the training. In response, the program team revised the training materials a second time and increased liaison responsibilities so that opinion leaders could acquire the skills necessary to have safer sex conversations with their peers.

Another program implementation issue that occurred was that, on occasion, the project team would lose contact with opinion leaders. Sometimes this was because an opinion leader had been sent to jail or had switched to working on the streets. These factors made the team think carefully about how these men's circumstances and life experiences could affect their ability to participate in the intervention and its evaluation. The team found no easy solutions to these challenges.

What were the end results of the adapted POL program? As was described in Figure 2–12, an evaluation was conducted using similar procedures to that of the original POL evaluation. Evaluation results showed that in two of the three bars where the program was conducted, men self-reported large decreases in rates of paid, unprotected anal and oral sex (Miller et al., 1998). Notably, in the two more successful bars, opinion leaders reported a greater sense of "ownership" of the intervention, participated more enthusiastically, developed greater camaraderie among themselves, and expressed greater motivation to be effective than participants at the third bar (Miller, 2003).

For further information about the original POL, including how to obtain program materials and training in POL implementation, see http://www.effectiveinterventions.org/interventions/POL.cfm, a Web page of the Centers for Disease Control and Prevention-sponsored Diffusion of Effective Behavioral Interventions (DEBI) Project.

**Standard 4.** Health care organizations must offer and provide language assistance services, including bilingual staff and interpreter services, at no cost to each patient/consumer with limited English proficiency at all points of contact, in a timely manner during all hours of operation.

**Standard 5.** Health care organizations must provide to patients/consumers in their preferred language both verbal offers and written notices informing them of their right to receive language assistance services.

**Standard 6.** Health care organizations must assure the competence of language assistance provided to limited English proficient patients/consumers by interpreters and bilingual staff. Family and friends should not be used to provide interpretation services (except on request by the patient/consumer).

**Standard 7.** Health care organizations must make available easily understood patient-related materials and post signage in the languages of the commonly encountered groups or groups represented in the service area.

**Figure 3-1 National Standards for Culturally and Linguistically Appropriate Services (CLAS) in Health Care: Language access services (OMH, 2001, pp. 10–13).**

service provision. Ultimately, limited access to services and poor communication between providers and clients can contribute to undesirable behavioral and health status outcomes among a program's target population.

## Improving Language Access

As was discussed in Section 1 (see especially Figure 1–3), the U.S. Office of Minority Health (OMH) has responded to the health care-related needs of persons with limited English proficiency (LEP) by issuing four language access service standards within its 14 *National Standards for Culturally and Linguistically Appropriate Services in Health Care (CLAS)* (OMH, 2001). These four standards are shown in Figure 3–1.

In addressing language access issues, is important to bear in mind that although agency staff may be bilingual, they may not be familiar with relevant technical terminology in both English and their native language. Thus, bilingual staff should be properly trained in technical terminology in the language or languages in which they will be interacting with clients (Grantmakers in Health, 2005).

In addition, as is reflected in CLAS Standard 4, friends and family should not be used to provide interpretation services for HIV testing, counseling, or medical care appointments, except per the specific request of the patient or client. Use of a friend or family may compromise a client's right to privacy, result in psychological trauma to the interpreter (especially if he or she is a child of the client), and lead to withholding of information by clients, misinterpretations, and misunderstandings. Professional interpreters or well-trained bilingual staff should be used instead (Grantmakers in Health, 2005).

Whether it is bilingual staff or professional interpreters who provide services in diverse languages, it is important to be aware that people who "speak the same language" may use distinct geographic or social dialects. For example, Puerto Ricans, Mexicans, and Colombians speak dialects of Spanish that differ somewhat with respect to pronunciation, vocabulary, and even grammar. To avoid misunderstandings, it is important to be aware of the geographic and social backgrounds of program clients and to ensure that service providers can understand and use the same language varieties.

It is also important to bear in mind that not all persons use a *spoken language* as their primary language. For example, among persons with hearing loss in the United States, a subset consider themselves to be members of the *Deaf community* (with a capital "D"). The U.S. Deaf community is a distinct cultural group, with a common history that is tied to the founding of schools for deaf children beginning in the early 1800s. The group also has its own language, a *gestural* or *signed language* called

# 3-3    Barriers to HIV Prevention Among Persons With Hearing Loss

Did you know that people with hearing loss are disproportionately affected by the HIV/AIDS epidemic? About 10% of the U.S. population has some degree of hearing loss. Research estimates that the HIV prevalence among this population is 5%, compared to 3% in the general population (NIH, 2002). Hearing loss also can be a symptom of AIDS-associated illnesses, as well as a side-effect of HIV treatment medication.

Yael Bat-Chava and colleagues from the New York University School of Medicine understood the importance of educating deaf and hard of hearing persons about HIV/AIDS risk, and educating HIV+ persons about the risk of hearing loss. Together with colleagues from the City University of New York Graduate Center and the Gay, Lesbian, and Straight Education Network (GLSEN), the research team set out to learn more about the barriers to HIV prevention faced by people with hearing loss in New York State (Bat-Chava et al., 2005).

Previous research about **deaf people** had shown that:

- Deaf people tend to have less knowledge of how HIV is transmitted and prevented than hearing persons (Gaskins, 1999).
- Persons who were born deaf and attended residential schools for the deaf tend to have the lowest levels of such knowledge (Heuttel & Rothstein, 2001).
- The greatest barriers to HIV/AIDS education among deaf people are related to language issues. Most HIV prevention and treatment materials are written at an eighth grade reading level. This presents a problem to many people who were deafened before the age of 3 and communicate by means of American Sign Language (ASL). On average, this group reads at a fourth grade level (Campbell, 1999; Joseph, 1993).
- Deaf people's access to medical care (both prevention- and treatment-related) is complicated by fears about loss of confidentiality. Professional interpreters are often not trusted, and when family members or friends serve as interpreters, privacy concerns prevent patients from discussing sensitive issues concerning personal HIV risks and prevention (Steinberg et al., 1999).

In contrast to deaf populations, there has been little research on the HIV prevention-related needs of **hard of hearing people** who used spoken English and lip reading to communicate. To learn more about the HIV/AIDS prevention-related needs of *both* deaf and hard of hearing persons, Bat-Chava and colleagues conducted focus groups and interviews with 134 deaf and hard of hearing people. Study participants included residents of four cities across New York State (New York City, Albany, Buffalo, and Rochester). Participants ranged in age from 15 to 76 years old and represented diverse ethnic backgrounds and sexual orientations. Several participants were also HIV-positive.

Findings from this study indicated that **deaf participants** had low levels of HIV/AIDS knowledge and faced several key barriers to learning more about this topic. Specifically, the adult deaf signers in the study:

- Had not been prepared by their schooling to understand messages about HIV/AIDS in the popular media.
- Had limited English literacy skills, making it difficult to read captioning on television or videos.
- Preferred visual educational materials and delivery formats that did not include large amounts of text.
- Perceived professional or informal interpreters to be a threat to their privacy in medical encounters, including HIV testing and counseling sessions.

**Hard of hearing participants**, by contrast, had a strong understanding of HIV/AIDS and how to protect themselves. They were proficient in English and had, on average, higher education levels than deaf study participants. This group *preferred* written HIV/AIDS educational materials. Notably, the two HIV+ hard of hearing participants in the study had lost their hearing as a result of AIDS-related illnesses—yet neither had been promptly referred for appropriate audiology (hearing-related) follow-up services.

**Both deaf and hard of hearing participants** reported that physicians and medical institutions were not prepared to communicate effectively with them. Many participants felt stigmatized for their hearing loss. In some cases, people pretended to understand material that was actually incomprehensible to them, resulting in further risk of miscommunication.

Based on these findings, Bat-Chava and colleagues offered the following recommendations for HIV/AIDS prevention services for deaf and hard of hearing persons:

1. Health care providers should be educated about the communication needs of deaf and hard of hearing persons and offer accommodations that foster the most effective communication possible.
2. HIV/AIDS education should be offered in sign language for deaf persons, preferably conducted in small groups led by deaf peer educators. For hard of hearing persons, more written materials should be developed.
3. All HIV test sites should offer professional ASL interpreter services. For facilities in locations with larger deaf populations that use ASL, an HIV counselor who is fluent in ASL should be on staff.
4. Information on HIV/AIDS-related hearing loss (due to disease or medication) should be made available to all persons with HIV. In addition, HIV+ patients should be screened for audiological disorders and referred to appropriate treatment services as needed.

As of January 2007, the New York State Department of Health AIDS Institute makes available a free pamphlet entitled "Clinician's guide to working with patients who are deaf and hard of hearing" (2005). For an order form, see http://www.hivguidelines.org/Public/Content.aspx?PageID=6#clinguide.

*American Sign Language (ASL)* that developed from French Sign Language, not from English. Not all persons who have profound hearing loss or consider themselves "deaf" use ASL; and not all persons who use ASL have profound hearing loss or consider themselves "deaf." Although it is not known how many primary users of ASL or other signed languages there are in the United States today, a recent analysis of available data concluded that up to 500,000 people in the United States used a signed language at home as of 1972 (Mitchell et al., 2006). A variety of interpreting services and other resources are available to facilitate effective communication with persons who have hearing loss, including those who use ASL (NY State Dept. of Health, 2005). A discussion of the barriers to HIV prevention among persons with hearing loss is provided in Tale 3–3.

Sometimes, despite an agency's best wishes or intentions, no one is available to communicate with a client in his or her preferred language. Agencies can take several steps to prepare for such encounters and help to put staff and clients more at ease in what are unquestionably challenging and stressful situations. First, agencies can prepare lists of key words and phrases in clients' languages, provide these lists to staff, and train staff to pronounce the items correctly. Second, agencies can train staff in how to appropriately manage situations in which language barriers exist. For example, often there is a tendency to shout or speak overly slowly, which can increase communication difficulties and tensions. Acknowledging the language barrier at the outset of the interaction, using grammatically simple sentences, a calm and clear voice, and appropriate gestures, and drawing pictures can all help to facilitate communication.

In addition to taking into account clients' spoken or signed languages, it is important to make available appropriate translations of written program materials for clients of diverse language backgrounds. One key challenge is to develop materials that are appropriate for groups that use different dialects of a single language (as mentioned earlier). Another challenge is to develop more pictorial materials (e.g.,

Strategies for Making Written Materials Accessible to Low-Literacy Populations (IMPACT Project, 2002; Zimmerman et al., 1996)

| Component of Materials | Strategies |
| --- | --- |
| Design and Layout | ■ Communicate a single message with each illustration.<br>■ Limit the number of concepts and pages in the material.<br>■ Leave plenty of empty space, to make the material easier to follow.<br>■ Make the material interactive (e.g., by including simple question/answer formats).<br>■ Arrange messages (e.g., condom use steps) in a sequence that is most logical to the audience, and number the steps of the sequence.<br>■ Include culturally appropriate illustrations that convey key messages—for example, images of people who look like members of your target population (see also later). |
| Illustrations | ■ Use culturally appropriate hair and clothing styles, colors, objects, and symbols.<br>■ Include simple but realistic illustrations that portray people and objects as they occur in everyday life.<br>■ Illustrate objects in appropriate scale and context.<br>■ Use appropriate illustrative styles (e.g., drawings, cartoons, photos) that are acceptable and comprehensible to the target audience.<br>■ Use a positive approach that encourages and motivates the audience. |
| Text | ■ Choose a type style and size that are easy to read (i.e., at least 14-point font for regular text and larger font for titles).<br>■ Use uppercase and lowercase letters, instead of all capitals.<br>■ Use underlining or boldface for emphasis; avoid an italic style, as it is difficult to read.<br>■ Use short words (when possible) and keep sentences short.<br>■ Restate important information periodically to reinforce messages.<br>■ Test the readability of the text with members of the target population. |
| Piloting | ■ Pilot test materials for comprehensibility and appropriateness of design, illustrations, and text.<br>■ Incorporate resulting revisions before using materials. |

with photos, diagrams, etc.) for groups with limited literacy in any language (see later in this section).

The California Endowment (http://www.calendow.org) makes available, free of charge, a number of resources that can help health care and social service providers, administrators, and others to address language access issues successfully. For example, see the annotated bibliography of research literature by Jacobs et al. (2003); the guide for choosing and using a language agency by Roat (2003); and the language services resource guide by Sampson (2006).

## Strategies for Working With Low-Literacy Populations

The populations at highest risk for HIV infection tend to be members of marginalized communities (e.g., women of color; gay, lesbian, bisexual, and transgender persons; substance abusers; sex workers; migrant populations; and out-of-school youth). In many of these communities, low literacy rates are common, limiting the utility of existing written or text-based prevention materials (IMPACT Project, 2002). Should this be an issue for your program, you can use strategies in Table 3–2 to develop print materials that use visual aids or pictures.

Tool 3–5: Checklist for Developing Effective Print Materials for Low-Literacy Populations can help you to implement these recommendations.

## Additional Communication Barriers

Communication difficulties between staff and clients in HIV prevention contexts may result from more than differences in the specific language or dialect that is spoken (Scott et al., 2005). For example, different use of body language, such as gestures, posture, and eye contact, may lead to discomfort or misunderstanding in program contexts. Different norms concerning what topics my be appropriately discussed with whom, and what speaking styles are respectful or disrespectful in particular situations, may also lead to frustration or discontent among both program participants and staff.

Frontline staff should be trained to identify and address the full range of cross-cultural communication issues that may arise in service encounters. A number of helpful practitioner-focused resources and training programs have been developed for this purpose. Many are described in a series of publications produced by The California Endowment (e.g., see Gilbert et al., 2003a, 2003b, 2003c).

## RETAINING PROGRAM STAFF

*Staff retention* is a challenge that any agency might face at any time. However, HIV prevention programs face particularly serious staff retention challenges because of factors such as low pay, overwork, limited advancement opportunities, disconnect from the target population, and "burnout" from the ongoing stress of seeking to address overwhelming human needs in an environment of severely limited resources. There are a number of steps you can take to help address high rates of staff turnover and improve staff retention. These steps fall into a number of key (overlapping) areas including communication, training, support, feedback, and recognition and rewards.

## Communication

Communication is the key to making staff feel important and valued and can increase retention significantly. Strategies for improving communication with and among staff include (National Mentoring Partnership, 2003):

- Holding **in person meetings with all staff** periodically to provide opportunities to discuss program challenges and successes.
- Sending **e-mail updates to all program staff** on a regular basis. This will help them feel connected to a larger community, as well as provide an opportunity to share new information about program and agency activities, funding, and special events.
- Have the program manager or coordinator **meet with or call staff individually** once a month to ask about program successes and challenges, share new ideas and information, and remind staff of their responsibilities. Monthly contact is important, even if staff have worked in your program for a significant period of time.
- Send **individual thank you letters** to staff at least twice a year. This is another opportunity to reinforce how important staffs are, show appreciation for their individual accomplishments, and maintain open lines of communication.

It is important that communication with and among staff be in alignment with staff members' cultural norms and practices. In addition, all staff should be trained and encouraged to set an example for each other of how to communicate effectively by being sensitive speakers and listeners, attentive and responsive to the needs, values, and experiences of others.

## Training

Another primary way to retain staff is to ensure that they feel well-equipped to deliver the program and to address any conflicts, dilemmas, or stresses that may arise. On the one hand, this requires training on program goals, content, and methods, as well as on principles of cultural competence and cross-cultural communication. On the other hand, it also involves providing ongoing training for the substantive and emotional components of their roles as HIV prevention educators, instructors, or counselors (Brown, 1998). Substantive areas for this additional training include new developments in HIV disease and prevention, new teaching methods and counseling approaches, and new developments in cultural awareness and sensitivity. A key emotional area for training is how to deal with the stress of working with at-risk or HIV-infected clients in a climate of tremendous need and very limited resources.

It is also helpful to offer staff members incremental opportunities to use and improve new skills and competencies that they gain through training and on-the-job experience. For example, entry-level staff may be given increasing managerial responsibilities. Be sure to provide constructive guidance and feedback on their progress.

## Support

In addition to communication and training, other types of support can play an important role in helping staff deal with the challenges of HIV prevention work (Brown, 1998; National Mentoring Partnership, 2003). For example, informal staff social events help to build a sense of cohesiveness and community that can diffuse some of the stresses of daily prevention work. Taking the time both at such events and at staff meetings to thank staff, recognize the challenges they face, and share positive comments from program participants, fellow staff, funders, or community members can help validate their efforts and experiences.

It is also helpful to equip staff with written copies of agency policies and other resources concerning how to address conflicts, concerns, or crises. Staff should be encouraged to share concerns with others in appropriate and constructive ways. Some may need individual and/or group counseling to address the stresses that arise from their work activities. It is important to provide such resources or referrals to staff who need them, and not to embarrass, stigmatize, or penalize those who use them.

## Two-Way Feedback

In many ways, staff are the key to your program. They need to feel that others understand what an important role they play in program success. Asking for and incorporating staff input and feedback on program and activities and policies help create a sense of investment in and commitment to the program. Team meetings, periodic one-on-one staff reviews or interviews, written surveys, and anonymous "suggestion boxes" are examples of helpful ways to obtain staff input. It is also important to have a mechanism for sharing, discussing, and acting on this input. For example, a portion of every staff meeting might be devoted to a discussion of staff concerns and suggestions for action. Identification of next steps and roles and responsibilities for implementing those steps should always be a feature of those discussions (The After School Corporation, 2001; Lemansky, 1998).

Providing constructive feedback to staff on their roles and accomplishments is also central to staff retention (National Mentoring Partnership, 2003). Regularly scheduled one-on-one staff review or check-in sessions are ideal opportunities to discuss these topics.

## Recognition and Rewards

Staff need to be recognized and rewarded for their work, whether they are working for pay or as volunteers. There are a number of creative ways to do this. For example, you might hold an appreciation brunch or dinner with small gifts and entertainment, at which program directors and community members or clients share their appreciation for program staff. Additional ways are to offer periodic "thank you" gift cards to local restaurants or shops; have program participants create cards, poems, or drawings about and for their instructors or facilitators; and to publish a hardcopy or Web-based newsletter, with pictures, to thank staff publicly (Lemansky, 1998; National Mentoring Partnership, 2003).

As you plan how to train, support, and reward staff, do not forget to ask staff directly about their needs. You can use input from group meetings, individual interviews, or surveys to collect information from staff on factors such as:

- Actual staff roles and responsibilities (vs. what is written in their job descriptions).
- Skills necessary to succeed as a staff member.
- Level of staff experience and comfort with program content, methods, and target population.
- Staff fears, concerns, and expectations about their positions and activities.
- Staff perceptions of training and support needs and preferred formats.
- Staff availability (in light of their other responsibilities) to participate in training or support activities.
- What would make staff feel more appreciated for the work they do.

Across program settings, the specific staff retention challenges may vary, along with the best solutions. An in-depth look at staff retention among people who care for HIV+ hemophiliacs is provided in Tale 3–4. Tool 3–6: Staff Retention Checklist can help you to address staff retention issues in your own setting.

## PRACTICING CULTURALLY COMPETENT PROGRAM MANAGEMENT

### The Many Roles of Program Managers

No matter how well designed a program is, or how effective it has been in another setting, it will not be successful without good management (Card et al., 2001). Managing an HIV prevention program involves many tasks. Managers oversee the day-to-day operations of the program, ensure that it is adequately staffed, track resource use, and report on program delivery and outcomes to Executive Directors, boards, and funders. Many program managers also simultaneously serve as direct service providers (e.g., counselors or health educators), recruit program participants, and write grant proposals. Program managers also have important roles to play in promoting culturally competent program implementation, as they can influence agency-wide policies and practices and take the lead in establishing a program environment that recognizes and incorporates cultural diversity.

**TALE FROM THE FIELD**

## 3-4    Retaining HIV Health Care Professionals

When staff of HIV prevention programs decide to leave, there are consequences for many people. Losing staff is difficult for other program team members, who have to deal with personnel shortages and transition periods. It is also costly for the institution, which must invest heavily in training new staff members. In addition, when clients lose the care of a long-term staff person, they may have an increased feeling of vulnerability.

Clearly, staff retention is very important in HIV/AIDS organizations, so how can it be accomplished more effectively? That was the question that interested Dr. Larry Brown of Rhode Island Hospital. Together with colleagues from around the country (Ohio, Massachusetts, Pennsylvania, and Washington) Brown carried out a longitudinal (long-term) study of health care professionals working with HIV-positive hemophilia patients (Brown et al., 2002). The research team analyzed how staff retention (over a 4-year period) was related to a number of factors, including job stresses, job characteristics, job satisfaction, and opportunities for professional development.

The researchers surveyed health care professionals working with HIV+ patients at a representative set of 40 (out of 159) hemophilia treatment centers across the United States. They sent out 283 surveys, of which 213 (75%) were returned. Two years later, the researchers sent their first follow-up survey to the 213 respondents and learned that 194 were still working in HIV+ patient care centers. After another 2 years, a second follow-up survey was sent to the treatment centers to determine the employment status of the respondents. The surveys included questions related to job tasks, interactions with colleagues, and patient care. They also included questions about participation in educational trainings/meetings and an overall sense of job satisfaction. Using questions/answer scales from the Maslach Burnout Inventory (MBI), researchers classified those with high emotional ex-

haustion and low personal accomplishment scores as having "burnout."

In the initial survey, 7.4% of respondents were classified as burnt out. Yet by the time of the 2-year follow-up survey, respondents showed a lower burnout rate of 2.1%. For those who stayed in their jobs, the burnout rate had actually dropped. Despite the stress involved in caring for HIV-positive clients, provider burnout among those who remained in their positions was relatively low. Reported levels of emotional exhaustion and personal accomplishment appeared similar to those of other health care professionals.

What about those who left? More than one-third of the HIV care professionals who were initially surveyed left their positions during the 4-year study period. Study findings suggested that the most significant predictor of staff retention was a staff member's rating of *stress involving colleagues*—the greater the stress, the more likely the staff member would leave his or her HIV-related position. Married staff were also significantly more likely to remain in their positions than nonmarried staff.

Based on these findings and those from earlier studies, the researchers concluded that social support can have a crucial, protective impact on HIV care professionals' feelings of stress. What forms of social support might help? Although the data suggested that staff educational activities did not promote staff retention or job satisfaction, the researchers noted that if staff trainings focused on creating team relationships, they could be helpful in building a sense of social support. They also recommended regular meetings of all staff members to encourage interaction and conflict resolution. Overall, activities that improve staff relationships and enhance a sense of collegial support can contribute to staff retention in HIV prevention and care programs.

## Influencing Policies and Procedures

Program managers can influence policies and procedures that affect a program's ability to address the culturally related needs of program participants. Such policies and procedures may address (National CASA Association, 2005a, 2005b; OMH, 2001):

- Agency and program mission, vision, and goals.
- Agency physical facilities (e.g., accessibility to persons with disabilities, layout, decorations, etc.).
- Funding sources that are sought (or not sought).
- Staff and leadership composition, recruitment, and training requirements.
- Solicitation and incorporation of staff, client, and community input and feedback on program services and agency practices.
- Provision of interpreting services or other accommodations for program participants with limited English proficiency.
- Public relations activities and materials.
- Strategic planning to increase agency, program, and staff cultural competence.

## Setting an Example for Program Staff

Program managers can also set an example for how program staff should interact with clients and community members, by setting a tone in which diverse viewpoints are solicited, respected, and acted upon. For example, managers can model, through their own behavior, how to communicate effectively by being a sensitive speaker and listener, attentive and responsive to the needs, values, and experiences of others (National CASA Association, 2005b).

## Working With Program Participants

Even program managers who do not themselves deliver direct services can take steps to engage actively with program participants and use the insights they obtain to improve the cultural competence, effectiveness, and efficiency of service delivery. These steps include:

- **Observing**. Visit your program regularly, with advance notice to program staff.
- **Listening**. Talk to participants outside program sessions and solicit feedback on program activities.
- **Thinking**. Think about participant ideas and how they might be used to improve the program.
- **Acting**. Meet with program staff to discuss potential actions based on participant input.

## Supporting Positive Relationships With the Local Community

Program managers can also play a key role in establishing and maintaining positive relationships with the local community, including other service organizations, community leaders, residents, and local funders (Card et al., 2001). For example, during program implementation, program managers can share service information with other agencies to promote interagency client referrals and expand program recruitment. Managers can also meet with community leaders to discuss service offerings and address any concerns about their goals, content, or format. In addition, managers can invite local funders to attend program events and observe the program in action. These points of contact afford managers additional opportunities to obtain input on how the program can be refined to better address the cultural needs, values, and norms of its clients.

Tool 3–7: Culturally Competent Program Management Checklist can help program managers to use their unique positions to promote more culturally competent programming.

# REFERENCES

The After School Corporation (TASC). (2001). After-school toolbox. Promising practices: Staff retention model. Retrieved October 13, 2005, from http://www.tascorp.org/toolbox/promising_practices/staff_retention

Bat-Chava, Y., Martin, D., & Kosciw, J. G. (2005). Barriers to HIV/AIDS knowledge and prevention among deaf and hard of hearing people. *AIDS Care, 17*(5), 623–634.

The Body. (2004, June). Advancing prevention for all populations. Debunking the "model minority" myth: Prevention for Asians and Pacific Islanders. *AIDS Action Weekly Update Special Edition.* Retrieved September 27, 2005, from http://www.thebody.com/aac/update/jun25_04/api.html

Brach, C., & Fraser, I. (2000). Can cultural competency reduce racial and ethnic health disparities? A review and conceptual model. *Medical Care Research and Review, 57*(1), 181–217.

Brindis, C., & Davis, L. (1998). *Improving contraceptive access for teens. (Communities responding to the challenge of adolescent pregnancy prevention, Vol. IV).* Washington, DC: Advocates for Youth. Retrieved August 2, 2005, from http://www.advocatesforyouth.org/publications/communitiesresponding4.pdf

Brown, B. S. (1998). *HIV/AIDS and drug abuse treatment services—part B, literature review.* Bethesda, MD: National Institute on Drug Abuse (NIDA). Retrieved October 13, 2005, from http://www.drugabuse.gov/about/organization/DESPR/HSR/da-tre/BrownHIVPartB.html

Brown, L. K., Schultz, J. R., Forsberg, A. D., King, G., Kocik, S. M., & Butler, R. B. (2002). Predictors of retention among HIV/hemophilia health care professionals. *General Hospital Psychiatry, 24*(1), 48–54.

Brown-Peterside, P., Rivera, E., Lucy, D., Slaughter, I., Ren, L., Chiasson, M. A., et al. (2001). Retaining hard-to-reach women in HIV prevention and vaccine trials: Project ACHIEVE. *American Journal of Public Health, 91*(9), 1377–1379.

Butterfoss, F. D., Goodman, R. M., & Wandersman, A. (1996). Community coalitions for prevention and health promotion: Factors predicting satisfaction, participation, and planning. *Health Education Quarterly, 23*(1), 65–79.

Campbell, D. (1999). AIDS and the deaf community. *ADVANCE for Speech-Language Pathologists and Audiologists, 10*–11.

Card, J. J., Brindis, C., Peterson, J. L., & Niego, S. (2001). *Guidebook: Evaluating teen pregnancy prevention programs* (2nd ed.). Los Altos, CA: Sociometrics Corporation.

Castro, F. G., Barrera, M., & Martinez, C. (2004). The cultural adaptation of prevention interventions: Resolving tensions between fidelity and fit. *Prevention Science, 5*(1), 41–45.

Conner, R. F., Takahashi, L., Ortiz, E., Archuleta, E., Muniz, J., & Rodriguez, J. (2005). The Solaar HIV Prevention Program for gay and bisexual Latino men: Using social marketing to build capacity for service provision and evaluation. *AIDS Education and Prevention, 17*(4), 361–374.

The Florida Department of Health. (2004). Community health status and improvement planning terminology. Retrieved August 1, 2005, from http://www.doh.state.fl.us/planning_eval/CHAI/Resources/FieldGuide/6CommHealthStat us/CHSATerminology.htm

Fortier, J. P., Convissor, R., & Pacheco, G. (1999). *Assuring cultural competence in health care: Recommendations for national standards and an outcomes-focused research agenda.* Washington, DC: Department of Health and Human Services and Resources for Cross Cultural Health Care.

Gaskins, S. (1999). Special population: HIV/AIDS among the deaf and hard of hearing. *Journal of the Association of Nurses in AIDS Care, 10*(2), 75–78.

Gilbert, M. J. (Ed.). (2003a). *A manager's guide to cultural competence education for health care professionals.* Woodlands, CA: The California Endowment. Retrieved May 12, 2005, from http://www.calendow.org/reference/publications/pdf/cultural/TCE0217-2003_A_Managers_Gui.pdf

Gilbert, M. J. (Ed.). (2003b). *Principles and recommended standards for cultural competence education of health care professionals.* Woodlands, CA: The California Endowment. Retrieved January 16, 2006, from http://www.calendow.org/reference/publications/pdf/cultural/TCE0215-2003_Principles_and.pdf

Gilbert, M. J. (Ed.). (2003c). *Resources in cultural competence education for health care professionals*. Woodlands, CA: The California Endowment. Retrieved January 16, 2006, from http://www.calendow.org/reference/publications/pdf/cultural/TCE0218-2003_Resources_in_C.pdf

Grantmakers in Health. (2005, August). *In the right words: Addressing language and culture in providing health care*. San Francisco: Grantmakers in Health. Retrieved January 16, 2006, from http://www.calendow.org/reference/publications/pdf/cultural/TCE0811-2002_In_the_Right_W.pdf

Harris, S. K., Samples, C. L., Keenan, P. M., Fox, D. J., Melchiono, M. W., Woods, E. R., & the Boston HAPPENS Program. (2003). Outreach, mental health, and case management services: Can they help to retain HIV-positive and at-risk youth and young adults in care? *Maternal and Child Health Journal, 7*(4), 205–218.

Heuttel, K. L., & Rothstein, W. G. (2001). HIV/AIDS knowledge and information sources among deaf and hard of hearing college students. *American Annals for the Deaf, 146*(3), 280–286.

Implementing AIDS Prevention and Care (IMPACT) Project. (2002). *Developing materials on HIV/AIDS/STIs for low-literate audiences*. Washington, DC: Family Health International (FHI) and Program for Appropriate Technology in Health (PATH). Retrieved September 28, 2005, from http://www.fhi.org/NR/rdonlyres/e2q7um2s2ffrtcjeesnjqhrgrt4bqawhrjqfreh02z23rc71pxiuny3kekvsed41g3sn50crpua3jn/lowlitguide2.pdf

Jacobs, E. A., Agger-Gupta, N., Chen, A. H., Piotrowski, A., & Hardt, E. J. (2003). Language barriers in health care settings: An annotated bibliography of the research literature. Woodland Hills, CA: The California Endowment. Retrieved March 17, 2007, from http://www.calendow.org/reference/publications/pdf/cultural/TCE0801-2003_Language_Barri.pdf

Janz, N. K., Zimmerman, M. A., Wren, P. A., Israel, B. A., Freudenberg, N., & Carter, R. J. (1996). Evaluation of 37 AIDS prevention projects: Successful approaches and barriers to program effectiveness. *Health Education Quarterly, 23*(1), 80–97.

Jemmott, J. B., III, Jemmott, L. S., & Fong, G. T. (1992). Reductions in HIV risk-associated sexual behaviors among black male adolescents: Effects of an AIDS prevention intervention. *American Journal of Public Health, 83*(3), 372–377.

Jemmott, L. S., Jemmott, J. B., III, & McCaffree, K. (1995). *Be proud! Be responsible! Strategies to empower youth to reduce their risk for AIDS*. New York: Select Media.

Joseph, J. (1993). Peer education and the deaf community. *College Health, 41*(6), 264–266.

Kelly, J. A., Murphy, D. A., Sikkema, K. J., McAuliffe, T. L., Roffman, R. A., Solomon, L. J., et al. & The Community HIV Prevention Research Collaborative. (1997). Randomised, controlled, community-level HIV-prevention intervention for sexual-risk behaviour among homosexual men in US cities. *Lancet, 350*(9090), 1500–1505.

Kelly, J. A., St. Lawrence, J. S., Diaz, Y. E., Stevenson, L. Y., Hauth, A. C., Kalichman, S. C., et al. (1991). HIV risk behavior reduction following intervention with key opinion leaders of population: An experimental analysis. *American Journal of Public Health, 81*(2), 1483–1489.

Kelly, J. A., St. Lawrence, J. S., Stevenson, L. Y., Hauth, A. C., Kalichman, S. C., Diaz, Y. E., et al. (1992). Community AIDS/HIV risk reduction: The effects of endorsements by popular people in three cities. *American Journal of Public Health, 82*(11), 1483–1489.

Kennedy, M. G., Mizuno, Y., Hoffman, R., Baume, C., & Strand, J. (2000). The effect of tailoring a model HIV prevention program for local adolescent target audiences. *AIDS Education and Prevention, 12*(3), 225–238.

Lehman, S. (2002). *Recruitment and retention challenges in the evaluation of youth drop-in centers: using youth focus groups to generate solutions*. Presentation at 5th Annual Conference on AIDS Research in California. Retrieved October 10, 2005, from http://uarp.ucop.edu/CommDissem/PresentSource/65Lehman.pdf

Lemansky, F. (1998). *Part-time staff retention*. [Monograph.] North East, PA: Pennsylvania Action Research Network. Retrieved May 7, 2006, from http://www.pde.state.pa.us/able/lib/able/lfp/lfp981emansky.pdf

Miller, R. L. (2003). Adapting an evidence-based intervention: Tales of the Hustler Project. *AIDS Education and Prevention, 15*(Suppl A), 127–138.

Miller, R. L., Klotz, D., & Eckholdt, H. M. (1998). HIV prevention with male prostitutes and patrons of hustler bars: Replication of an HIV prevention intervention. *American Journal of Community Psychology, 26*(1), 97–131.

Mitchell, R. E., Young, T. A., Bachleda, B., & Karchmer, M. A. (2006). How many people use ASL in the United States? Why estimates need updating. *Sign Language Studies, 6*(3), 306–335.

National CASA Association. (2005a). Cultural competence in your program. Retrieved September 15, 2005, from http://www.casanet.org/program-management/diversity/cultural-competence.htm

National CASA Association. (2005b). Becoming culturally competent. Retrieved September 15, 2005, from http://permanent.access.gpo.gov/lps9890/lps9890/www.casanet.org/program-management/diversity/becomcul.htm

National Institutes of Health (NIH). (2002). HIV/AIDS statistics. Retrieved May 23, 2003, from http://www.niaid.nih.gov/factsheets/aidsstat.htm

National Mentoring Partnership. (2003). Sustaining and energizing your volunteers: Retention strategies for mentoring programs. Summary of best practices. *Retention Forum, 1*(2). Retrieved October 13, 2005, from http://www.mentoring.org/program_staff/files/retentionforum03.pdf

New York State Department of Health. (2005). Clinician's guide to working with patients who are deaf and hard of hearing [pamphlet]. [Note: As of January 25, 2007, copies are free of charge from the New York State Department of Health AIDS Institute; for an order form, see http://www.hivguidelines.org/Public/Content.aspx?PageID=6#clinguide]

Office of Minority Health (OMH), U.S. Department of Health and Human Services. (2001). *National standards for culturally and linguistically appropriate services in health care: Final report.* Washington, DC: OMH. Retrieved January 16, 2006, from http://www.omhrc.gov/assets/pdf/checked/finalreport.pdf

Ramirez-Valles, J., & Brown, A. U. (2003). Latinos' community involvement in HIV/AIDS: Organizational and individual perspectives on volunteering. *AIDS Education and Prevention, 15*(1 Suppl A), 90–104.

Roat, C. E. (2003). *How to choose and use a language agency: A guide for health and social service providers who wish to contract with language agencies.* Retrieved March 17, 2007, from http://www.calendow.org/reference/publications/pdf/cultural/TCE0220-2003_How_To_Choose_.pdf

Sampson, A. (2006). *Language services resource guide for health care providers.* Los Angeles, CA: National Health Law Program. Retrieved March 17, 2007, from http://www.calendow.org/reference/publications/pdf/cultural/ResourceGuideFinal.pdf

Santos, G., Puga, A. M., & Medina, C. (2004). HAART, adherence, and cultural issues in the US Latino community. *The AIDS Reader, 14*(10 Suppl), S26–S29.

Scott, K. D., Gilliam, A., & Braxton, K. (2005). Culturally competent strategies for women of color in the United States. *Health Care for Women International, 26*(1), 17–45.

Shin, H. B., & Bruno, R. (2003). Language use and English-speaking ability: 2000. *Census 2000 Brief, C2KBR-29,* 1–11. Retrieved June 18, 2005, from http://www.census.gov/prod/2003pubs/c2kbr-29.pdf

Steinberg, A. G., Lowe, R. C., & Sullivan, V. J. (1999). The diversity of consumer knowledge, attitudes, beliefs, and experiences: Recent findings. In I. W. Leigh (Ed.), *Mental health interventions and the Deaf community* (pp. 23–43). Washington, DC: Gallaudet University Press.

Sumartojo, E. (2000). Structural factors in HIV prevention: Concepts, examples, and implications for research. *AIDS, 14*(Suppl 1), S3–S10.

Villarruel, A .M., Jemmott, L. S., & Jemmott, J. B., III. (2005). Designing a culturally based intervention to reduce HIV sexual risk for Latino adolescents. *Journal of the Association of Nurses in AIDS Care, 16*(2), 23–31.

Villarruel, A. M., Jemmott, L. S., Jemmott, J. B., III, & Eakin, B. L. (2006a). Recruitment and retention of Latino adolescents to a research study: Lessons learned from a randomized clinical trial. *Journal for Specialists in Pediatric Nursing, 11*(4), 244–250.

Villarruel, A. M., Jemmott, L. S., Jemmott, J. B., III, & Eakin, B. L. (2006b). A randomized controlled trial testing an HIV prevention intervention for Latino youth. *Archives of Pediatrics and Adolescent Medicine, 160*(8), 772–777.

Wakefield, S. (2001). NYC HVTU sets standard for recruiting and retaining hard-to-reach women. *HIV Vaccines and the Community: The Community Advisory Board Bulletin, 2*(10), 1. Retrieved October 10, 2005, from http://www.hvtn.org/pdf/community/Bulletin11-01.pdf

Zimmerman, M. L., Newton, N., Frumin, L., & Wittet, S. (1996). *Developing health and family planning materials for low-literate audiences: A guide (rev. ed.).* Washington, DC: PATH. Retrieved September 29, 2005, from http://www.path.org/files/DC_Low_Literacy_Guide.pdf

# Tool 3-1 Matrix for Involving Community Leaders in Program Implementation[1]

It is important to think through how you will involve community leaders (e.g., community organizers or activists, leaders of places of worship, community elders, neighborhood committee members, and others who are respected in the community) in your program implementation efforts. The matrix below will help you do this.

To fill in the table below on your computer (using the file on the CD-ROM), click on the gray-shaded area in the box you would like to type in. (Note that the gray shading will not appear in printouts of this document.) Alternately, you may photocopy this tool (for your use only) and complete it by hand or typewriter.

| Name of Community Leader | Contact Information | Areas of Interest or Expertise | Possible Program Implementation Roles, e.g.: ■ Outreach worker for participant recruitment ■ Volunteer peer educator ■ Member of team that helps monitor program delivery |
|---|---|---|---|
|  |  |  |  |
|  |  |  |  |
|  |  |  |  |
|  |  |  |  |
|  |  |  |  |
|  |  |  |  |

[1] Adapted from Card, J. J., Brindis, C., Peterson, J. L., & Niego, S. (2001). *Guidebook: Evaluating teen pregnancy prevention programs* (2nd ed., Exercise 4.1). Los Altos, CA: Sociometrics Corporation.

# Tool 3-2 Participant Recruitment Checklist

When designing a recruitment plan for your HIV prevention program, consider the strategies listed in the table below. Place an "x" in the square box (□) next to the items that are of greatest relevance to your program. (To do this on your computer—using the file on your CD-ROM—use your cursor to click on the box. To remove an "x" from a box, click on the box again.) Then, for each item you select, identify the steps that will need to be taken and who will have responsibility for those steps. To type into the middle and far right columns, click on the gray-shaded area in the box you wish to type in. (Note that the gray shading will not appear in printouts of this document.)

| STRATEGIES | STEPS TO BE TAKEN | WHO IS RESPONSIBLE |
|---|---|---|
| □ Develop recruitment materials and outreach protocols.<br>  □ Include materials in all relevant languages.<br>  □ Review for culturally appropriate messages/images. | | |
| □ Disseminate written recruitment materials.<br>  □ Post fliers at sites frequented by your target population.<br>  □ Post ads in local newspapers, magazines, or online listserves. | | |
| □ Make presentations and host information booths at local community events (e.g., festivals, street fairs, PTA meetings). | | |
| □ Send outreach workers to meet with target groups. | | |
| □ Cross-market your program.<br>  □ Recruit among clients enrolled in other programs within your agency.<br>  □ Recruit among clients enrolled in other agencies' programs. | | |
| □ Hold an "open house."<br>  □ Invite community members to meet your staff.<br>  □ Provide information to publicize your program. | | |
| □ Set up a toll-free telephone number and Web site for easy initial contact with the program. | | |
| □ Provide age- and culturally appropriate incentives for program enrollment (e.g., T-shirts, gift cards, condoms, key chains). | | |
| □ Offer transportation, transportation vouchers, or child care services to reduce barriers to program participation. | | |
| □ Other (indicate:) | | |

# Tool 3-3 Participant Retention Checklist

When designing a participant retention plan for your program, consider the strategies listed in the table below. Place an "x" in the square box (□) next to the items that are of greatest relevance. (To do this on your computer—using the file on your CD-ROM—use your cursor to click on the box. To remove an "x" from a box, click on the box again.)

Then, for each item you select, identify the steps that will need to be taken and who will have responsibility for those steps. To type into the middle and right columns, click on the gray-shaded area in the box you wish to type in. (Note that the gray shading will not appear in printouts of this document.)

| STRATEGIES | STEPS TO BE TAKEN | WHO IS RESPONSIBLE |
|---|---|---|
| □ Provide transportation or transportation vouchers. | | |
| □ Make child care available for participants with young children. | | |
| □ Provide age- and culturally appropriate incentives (e.g., T-shirts, gift cards, a graduation certificate and ceremony for those who complete the program). | | |
| □ Provide counseling or make referrals to other services (e.g., for mental health, substance abuse, housing, employment, domestic violence, and other issues). | | |
| □ Plan appropriate social activities (e.g., holiday parties). | | |
| □ Make personalized contact (by phone, mail, e-mail, or in person, as appropriate), especially to participants who miss sessions. | | |
| □ Other *(indicate:)* | | |

# Tool 3-4 Worksheet for Responding to Target Population Needs

It is important to monitor your program as soon as implementation begins so that you can be aware of any issues, barriers, or needs among your target population that may adversely affect their program participation, service satisfaction, or outcomes. This worksheet will help you to summarize any issues that arise and brainstorm strategies for addressing them. (Be aware that some issues may cut across several rows or categories.)

To fill in the table below on your computer (using the file on the CD-ROM), click on the gray-shaded area in the box you would like to type in. (Note that the gray shading will not appear in printouts of this document.) Alternately, you may photocopy this tool (for your use only) and complete it by hand or typewriter.

| *I. LOGISTICAL BARRIERS TO PROGRAM PARTICIPATION* | | |
| --- | --- | --- |
| **Potential Issue** | **Specific Problem Noted** | **Strategies for Addressing the Problem** |
| a. Inaccessible program schedule (e.g., day of week, time of day, frequency of sessions) | | |
| b. Inaccessible program location (e.g., due to transportation problems, no accommodation for disabilities, etc.) | | |
| c. Fee is too high or insurance requirement cannot be met | | |
| d. Lack of child care | | |
| e. Lack of staff who speak clients' language(s) | | |
| f. Program materials assume too high a literacy level | | |
| g. Other *(indicate:)* | | |
| *II. PERCEIVED BARRIERS TO PROGRAM PARTICIPATION* | | |
| **Potential Issue** | **Specific Problem Noted** | **Strategies for Addressing the Problem** |
| a. Clients feel that the program is boring or not relevant to them | | |
| b. Clients are uncomfortable with staff | | |
| c. Clients feel that physical facilities are "unfriendly" | | |
| d. Clients are concerned about confidentiality issues | | |
| e. Clients fear being arrested or deported | | |
| f. Other *(indicate:)* | | |

| III. OTHER PROBLEMS WITH THE CULTURAL COMPETENCE OF THE PROGRAM | | |
| --- | --- | --- |
| **Potential Issue** | **Specific Problem Noted** | **Strategies for Addressing the Problem** |
| a. The program is not targeting the right range or level of HIV risk factors | | |
| b. The program is not developmentally appropriate | | |
| c. The program's content or delivery formats are not culturally appropriate | | |
| d. The vocabulary and images in program materials are not culturally appropriate | | |
| e. The staff are not adequately prepared to work with the target population | | |
| f. Participant recruitment or retention strategies are not culturally appropriate | | |
| g. Other *(indicate:)* | | |

## Tool 3-5 Checklist for Developing Effective Print Materials for Low-Literacy Populations[1]

This checklist will help you to develop materials for low-literacy populations. Place an "x" in the square box (☐) as you address each item. (To do this on your computer—using the file on your CD-ROM—use your cursor to click on the box. To remove an "x" from a box, click on the box again.)

## 1. Design/Layout

☐ Communicate a single message with each illustration.

☐ Limit the number of concepts and pages in the material.

☐ Make the material interactive (e.g., by including simple question/answer formats).

☐ Leave plenty of empty space, to make the material easier to follow.

☐ Arrange messages (e.g., condom use steps) in an order that is most logical to the audience.

☐ Number the steps of the sequence.

☐ Include culturally appropriate illustrations (e.g., images of people who look like members of your target population) that support key messages. (See also #2.)

## 2. Illustrations

☐ Use culturally appropriate hair and clothing styles, colors, objects, and symbols.

☐ Include realistic yet simple images that portray people and objects as they occur in everyday life.

☐ Illustrate objects in appropriate scale and context.

☐ Use appropriate illustrative styles (e.g., drawings, cartoons, photos) that are acceptable and comprehensible to the audience.

☐ Use positive images that encourage and motivate the audience.

## 3. Text

☐ Choose a type style and size that are easy to read (e.g., a 14-point font for regular text and larger sizes for titles and subtitles).

☐ Use uppercase and lowercase letters, instead of all capitals.

☐ Use underlining or boldface for emphasis; avoid an italic style.

☐ Use short, clear, comprehensible words and sentences.

☐ Restate important information periodically to reinforce messages.

## 4. Piloting

☐ Pilot test materials for comprehensibility and appropriateness of design, illustrations, and text.

☐ Incorporate resulting revisions before using materials.

---

[1] The content of this tool was derived from: (a) Implementing AIDS Prevention and Care (IMPACT) Project. (2002). *Developing materials on HIV/AIDS/STIs for low-literate audiences.* Washington, DC: Family Health International (FHI) and Program for Appropriate Technology in Health (PATH). Retrieved September 8, 2005, from http://www.fhi.org/NR/rdonlyres/ e2q7um2s2ffrtcjeesnjqhrgrt4bqawhrjqfreho2z23rc7lpxiuny3kekvsed4lg3sn5ocrpua3jn/lowlitguide2.pdf (b) Zimmerman, M. L., Newton, N., Frumin, L., & Wittet, S. (1996). *Developing health and family planning materials for low-literate audiences: A guide, revised edition.* Washington, DC: PATH. Retrieved September 29, 2005, from http://www.path.org/files/DC_Low_Literacy_Guide.pdf

# Tool 3-6 Staff Retention Checklist

A staff retention strategy for your HIV prevention program might include some or all of the elements listed in the table below.

Place an "x" in the square box (□) next to the items that are of greatest relevance to your program and agency. (To do this on your computer—using the file on your CD-ROM—use your cursor to click on the box. To remove an "x" from a box, click on the box again.) To type into the "Notes" column, click on the gray-shaded area in the box you wish to type in. (Note that the gray shading will not appear in printouts of this document.)

| STRATEGIES AND ACTIVITIES | NOTES |
|---|---|
| □ **Communication Strategies**<br> □ Hold periodic in person meetings with all staff.<br> □ Send regular e-mail updates to all staff.<br> □ Hold monthly individual meetings or calls with staff. | |
| □ **Training Strategies**<br> □ Offer program goals, content, and methods trainings.<br> □ Offer cultural competence and cross-cultural communication trainings.<br> □ Offer trainings on HIV prevention issues.<br> □ Offer trainings on emotional aspects (e.g., stress) of HIV prevention programming. | |
| □ **Support Strategies**<br> □ Provide staff with written copies of program policies.<br> □ Hold informal staff social events.<br> □ Equip staff with resources on how to address conflicts, concerns, or crises.<br> □ Offer individual and/or group counseling to address work-related stresses.<br> □ Thank and share positive comments about staff at staff meetings. | |
| □ **Feedback Strategies**<br> □ Elicit staff input via team meetings, staff reviews, surveys, and "suggestion boxes."<br> □ Discuss staff ideas at staff meetings, in casual conversations, and via e-mail.<br> □ Act on staff input in current program cycle and in future program and evaluation planning.<br> □ Provide constructive feedback via regularly scheduled one-on-one staff check-in meetings.<br> □ Offer opportunities for staff to use and improve skills. | |
| □ **Recognition and Rewards**<br> □ Hold an appreciation brunch or dinner.<br> □ Offer periodic "thank you" gift cards to local restaurants or shops.<br> □ Have program clients create cards, poems, or drawings for their instructors or facilitators.<br> □ Send individual thank you letters to staff annually.<br> □ Publish a hardcopy or Web-based newsletter, with pictures, that thanks staff publicly. | |

# Tool 3-7 Culturally Competent Program Management Checklist[1]

This checklist will help you ensure that your program management practices are promoting culturally competent programming.

Place an "x" in the square box (□) as you complete each item. (To do this on your computer—using the file on your CD-ROM—use your cursor to click on the box. To remove an "x" from a box, click on the box again.) To type into the "Notes" column, click on the gray-shaded area in the box you wish to type in. (Note that the gray shading will not appear in printouts of this document.)

□ **1. Use your influence as a manager (or encourage your manager) to ensure that program and agency policies and practices are sensitive to and appropriate for the needs, assets, and preferences of the cultural groups that you serve. To do so, first ask yourself:**

| QUESTIONS | NOTES |
|---|---|
| □ Is there a commitment to inclusiveness in your agency's and department's mission and vision? | |
| □ Is there a commitment to recruiting culturally diverse staff who reflect the composition of the target population and local community? | |
| □ Is training in cultural competence provided on an ongoing basis to all staff (including volunteers, managers, etc.)? | |
| □ Are physical facilities inviting to people of various cultures? Are they accessible to people with physical disabilities? | |
| □ Are staff and client grievance and suggestion procedures accessible, fairly applied, and made widely known to staff and clients? | |
| □ Is funding sought and obtained from agencies whose values are consistent with cultural diversity and tolerance? | |
| □ Are public relations activities and materials appropriate for culturally diverse audiences? | |
| □ Are bilingual staff or appropriate interpreting services available for clients with limited English proficiency? | |
| □ Do strategic planning activities take into account a commitment to diversity and inclusiveness? | |

---

[1] The content of this tool was derived in part from: (a) National CASA Association. (2005a). Cultural competence in your program. Retrieved September 15, 2005, from http://www.casanet.org/program-management/diversity/cultural-competence.htm (b) National CASA Association. (2005b). Becoming culturally competent. Retrieved September 15, 2005, from http://permanent.access.gpo.gov/lps9890/lps9890/www.casanet.org/program-management/diversity/becomcul.htm

☐ **2. Create an environment in which diverse staff viewpoints are solicited, respected, and acted on. The following practices can help you do so:**

| PRACTICES | NOTES |
|---|---|
| ☐ Meet regularly with staff, in groups and one-on-one. | |
| ☐ Ensure that all staff, and not just the most vocal ones, have an opportunity to participate in group discussions. | |
| ☐ Set an example of how to be a good communicator:<br>☐ Be aware of your own past experiences in similar communicative situations.<br>☐ Be sensitive to the experiences of other speakers and listeners in similar communicative situations.<br>☐ Confront your own stereotypes.<br>☐ Ask questions, and be willing to learn about others.<br>☐ Teach others about yourself.<br>☐ Acknowledge your own thoughts and worries.<br>☐ Be aware of others' moods and concerns.<br>☐ Be aware of emotional messages that words may convey.<br>☐ Ask for clarification of the meaning of emotionally charged messages. | |
| ☐ Make available an anonymous "suggestion box." | |

☐ **3. Engage with program participants, even if you are not a direct service provider. Strategies for doing this include:**

| STRATEGIES | NOTES |
|---|---|
| ☐ Visit the program regularly to observe staff and participants in action. *(Note: first consult with program staff about appropriate opportunities for doing this.)* | |
| ☐ Talk with program participants outside program sessions and solicit their feedback on program activities. | |
| ☐ Think about how to incorporate participant ideas into program improvement efforts. | |
| ☐ Meet with program staff to discuss potential actions based on participant input. | |

☐ **4. Work effectively with community members. Strategies for doing this include:**

| STRATEGIES | NOTES |
|---|---|
| ☐ Share service information with other agencies to promote interagency client referrals and expand program recruitment. | |
| ☐ Meet with community leaders and members at community forum events or agency "open houses" to discuss program offerings and any concerns the community may have about the goals, content, or format of your programming. | |
| ☐ Attend community events to promote the program through information booths or presentations. | |
| ☐ Invite local funders to attend program events and observe the program in action. *(Note: first consult with program staff about appropriate opportunities for doing this.)* | |

# Culturally Competent Program Evaluation

## OVERVIEW

*Culturally competent program evaluation* involves being aware of the cultural norms, attitudes, and beliefs of the communities your program serves and incorporating them into all aspects of assessment of program processes and outcomes. Involving program stakeholders (including staff, community members, and representatives of the program's target population) in all evaluation activities, from design to data collection, analysis, and reporting, can help to ensure that this happens. This section will cover the nine topics below.

## 1. Integrating Community Leaders Into Culturally Competent Program Evaluation

Involving community leaders in program evaluation helps promote a culturally competent evaluation. Community leaders can help to set evaluation priorities, review proposed methods and instruments, interpret data, develop recommendations, and disseminate findings. They can also promote involvement of other community members in the evaluation.

## 2. Protecting Human Subjects

A *human subject* is an individual whose physical or behavioral responses are studied for the purposes of a research project. Because evaluation is a type of research, program participants (and any other community members who provide evaluation data) are considered human subjects. HIV prevention program evaluation commonly involves collection of information from human subjects through discussions, interviews, surveys, medical exams, or case file reviews. Evaluators must inform all study participants of their rights and obtain their express permission to take part in a study. A culturally competent evaluation pays particular attention to participants' culturally specific needs with respect to this permission and participants' right to privacy.

## 3. Distinguishing Process Evaluation From Outcome Evaluation

A *process evaluation* assesses the program as implemented versus what was planned. As such, it can document the services delivered, population reached, and resources used, as well as participant and staff satisfaction of the program as delivered. An outcome evaluation, in contrast, focuses on whether a program had the desired impact, for whom, and under what circumstances. In choosing an evaluation type, consider the questions you and your stakeholders (e.g., agency, community, funders) want answered, the status of your program planning and implementation efforts, and the available resources.

## 4. Conducting a Culturally Competent Process Evaluation

A culturally competent process evaluation takes into account program participant, staff, and community needs and beliefs, as it assesses the program as it was actually implemented versus what was planned. Conducting a culturally competent process evaluation involves formulating research questions, selecting data collection and analysis methodologies, and interpreting findings in a manner consistent with local cultural norms.

## 5. Using Process Evaluation Results

Process evaluation results can provide direction for program improvement, inform program resource allocation, support accountability to funders, enhance community standing, help assess outcome evaluation readiness, and inform outcome evaluation findings. They can also suggest areas for improvement with respect to the program's cultural competence. The results should be disseminated to project stakeholders and used to build an action plan for future programming efforts.

## 6. Assessing Readiness for Culturally Competent Outcome Evaluation

To assess your program and agency readiness for a culturally competent outcome evaluation, it is important to consider: (a) strength of your program design; (b) strength of your program implementation; (c) accessibility of program participants and a potential comparison group; (d) availability of resources; and (e) potential for involving program stakeholders in evaluation activities. Assessing all of these factors can help you make an informed decision concerning outcome evaluation readiness.

## 7. Conducting a Culturally Competent Outcome Evaluation

Guided by a set of research questions, a culturally competent outcome evaluation identifies and measures an HIV prevention program's impact and whether it has achieved its goals and objectives with respect to changes in the target population. Culturally competent outcome evaluation requires early planning; identification of indicators, measurement methods, and measurement instruments; development and execution of appropriate data collection, analysis, and interpretation procedures; and involvement of stakeholders in all of these activities, to help ensure that the evaluation findings will ultimately be helpful to the local community. An appropriate outside evaluator is often key to ensuring the successful implementation of an outcome evaluation.

## 8. Reporting Outcome Evaluation Findings

Before reporting process or outcome evaluation results widely, program staff and other key stakeholders, including community members, should work together to review the findings and decide how and with whom to share them. It is important to identify appropriate audiences, mediums, and formats for the results; make explicit

links between results and community needs; explain negative findings; work to ensure that results will not negatively impact community empowerment; and connect
findings to concrete action.

## 9. Using Outcome Evaluation Findings

Outcome evaluation results can inform program resource decisions, provide accountability to funders, enhance program standing in the community, aid in secur-
ing new funding, inform best practices in HIV prevention, and demonstrate links
between culturally competent programming and positive program outcomes. In addition, you can use outcome evaluation findings to develop an action plan to improve
your HIV prevention programming efforts.

   To help make the concept of culturally competent evaluation more concrete, a
perspective on culturally competent program evaluation in American Indian communities is provided in Tale 4–1.

## INTEGRATING COMMUNITY LEADERS INTO CULTURALLY COMPETENT PROGRAM EVALUATION

### Why Involving Community Leaders in Program Evaluation Is Important

As was indicated in Sections 2 and 3, a community leader is anyone whom group
members identify as their representative or as someone they respect. Community
leaders can help you define evaluation goals and methods that are aligned well with
the community's cultural values, norms, and beliefs. This will increase the likelihood
that the evaluation measures what is relevant to the community, produces data that
reflect what you intended to measure, and yields findings that help you to make
program changes and advocate for additional resources to address key client and
community needs.

### Identifying Community Leaders

As was discussed in Sections 2 and 3, community leaders can be identified through
a variety of channels and venues. It is important to remember that members of any
community (e.g., African Americans, transgendered individuals, men-who-have-
sex-with-men) have diverse cultural affiliations, based on dimensions such as gender, age, ethnicity, immigration status, and sexual orientation. So not everyone in a
particular community will agree on who the respected leaders are (Butterfoss et al.,
1996). You should therefore be sure to identify leaders within the various subgroups
of your community.

### Community Leaders as Resources for Program Evaluation

Community leaders can contribute to the cultural competence of an evaluation in
a number of key ways. For example, they can (Butterfoss et al., 1996; King et al.,
2004; Miller, 2003):

- Identify community values, attitudes, and beliefs that should to be taken into
  consideration in decisions about evaluation goals and methods.
- Help set evaluation priorities and questions.
- Serve on a steering committee to oversee the evaluation process.
- Review proposed evaluation methods and instruments and provide feedback
  on their appropriateness for program participants' cultural backgrounds.

# 4-1    Culturally Competent Evaluation in Indian Country

What does it mean to evaluate a prevention program in a *culturally competent* manner? In broad terms, a culturally competent evaluation involves (a) an appreciation for cultural differences; (b) a quest for expanding cultural knowledge, and (c) an effort to build relationships with those groups being evaluated. Using research methodologies that are in line with the practices of the groups being evaluated is another characteristic of a culturally competent evaluation effort (LaFrance, 2004). Program evaluators must realize they can never fully know every cultural detail of the group(s) involved in a program evaluation. However, they can and should strive for *greater cultural understanding* of these groups—not only as an end result of an evaluation but also as part of the evaluation process itself.

Joan LaFrance has conducted culturally competent evaluations in her work with American Indian and Alaska Native tribes and organizations. Her efforts to more fully understand the cultural concepts of *tribal sovereignty* and *tribal self-determination* have had a profound impact on her evaluation projects in Indian Country. (*Indian Country* refers to tribal nations and Alaskan native communities that recognize a common homeland where they live in community with one another.)

LaFrance's work helps illustrate why sovereignty is a critical concept to understand when developing an HIV program evaluation that is culturally appropriate for Native American groups. Sovereign tribal lands are separate governmental units, often run by a general council of adult citizens in a tribe as well as an elected tribal council. These lands have separate, distinct processes of governance that impact how HIV (and other) prevention programs are designed, implemented, and evaluated. It is through this concept of *sovereignty* that tribal governance and independent nationhood have come to be recognized, and both self-respect and respect for others have been built.

At the same time, a history of exploitation and self-serving research by outsiders has led Native American community members to be wary of projects that may benefit only the researcher and

not the local community. Researchers and evaluators need to be aware of this historical legacy and sensitive to the potential impact of their work in these communities.

Evaluators also need to learn culturally appropriate ways to work with tribal communities. For example, because these groups are often engaged in efforts to protect their land and self-governance rights, they may be reluctant to have evaluation results publicized that negatively portray their community. Evaluators need to work closely with key community members in the evaluation process; this will increase the likelihood of obtaining valid and useful findings and, in turn, potentially strengthen the rights of native communities.

When designing and implementing evaluations, program evaluators also need to respect local values and "ways of knowing." For example, in most Western research, "evidence" and knowledge tend to be based on *empirical research*—that is, on research involving actual observations and experiences with a subject. In contrast, in some native cultures, evidence and knowledge come from *trust-based mutual understandings* that evolve within relationships. In another example, although mainstream U.S. culture has historically valued individualism and mobility, native tribes often value a *sense of place*—a profound sense of connection to community and location. This value includes an understanding of the self as part of nature and nature as a part of the self. This value may translate into personal sacrifice in the name of the reservation. Thus a tribe may define a successful prevention program by the degree to which the program contributes to the larger tribal goal of restoring and preserving their land. HIV prevention programs and their evaluations must be seen as efforts that will contribute to the strengthening of the community and its ability to maintain tribal land.

These examples also illustrate how the tribal value of *self-determination* can have a significant impact on evaluation activities. Culturally competent evaluation efforts should engage indigenous peoples in setting the research agenda, choosing and designing the evaluation methods, and ensuring that the entire evaluation effort respects their sense of place, values, and culture.

Without a strong understanding of Indian Country values, program evaluators may very well misperceive a program's goals, content or criteria for success. The end result may be an evaluation report with unrepresentative data and potentially serious consequences (e.g., program cutbacks, stereotyping, and further misunderstandings among groups). In contrast, culturally competent evaluations can lead to more accurate analyses of program delivery and outcomes. They also increase the likelihood of yielding results that can be put to work to improve HIV prevention programs and policies.

What, specifically, can evaluators do to work more in more culturally competent ways with American Indian tribes and other cultural groups that have been traditionally marginalized or oppressed? First, they can demonstrate respect for the program as originally envisioned by local leaders and community members. They also can help program providers and participants to feel a sense of partnership in the evaluation process. In addition, evaluators can help communities to build capacity for conducting their own evaluations, thereby increasing community resources and autonomy. It is also important for evaluators to maximize the potential relevance of the evaluation findings for the populations being studied. Finally, evaluators should strive to give back to communities throughout the evaluation process, by helping them with fund development efforts, training, and obtaining a voice with outside audiences. Balancing the various considerations involved in culturally competent evaluation is not always easy, but it has the potential to not only improve HIV prevention services but also strengthen communities and intercommunity relationships.

- Interpret evaluation data in a manner consistent with community values.
- Develop recommendations and an action plan based on evaluation findings.
- Help disseminate evaluation findings to other community members.

Community leaders can also encourage program participants and other community members (such as citizen volunteers, graduate students from nearby universities, or local businesses) to participate in evaluation activities, which is vital to the success of the evaluation.

Tool 4–1: Who Can Help You Carry Out a Culturally Competent Evaluation? can facilitate your identification and involvement of various parties, including community leaders, in program evaluation efforts.

## PROTECTING HUMAN SUBJECTS

### What Is Human Subjects Protection?

A *human subject* is an individual whose physical or behavioral responses are studied for the purposes of a research project (Office for Human Research Protections, 2005). Because evaluation is a type of research, program participants (and any other community members who provide evaluation-related data) are considered human subjects. Evaluators collect information (or *data*) from human subjects by interacting with them in a discussion or interview, having them complete a survey, commissioning a medical examination (such as tests of blood, urine, or vaginal fluids), or reviewing a case file. Some of the information that evaluators collect may be very sensitive, particularly when it is about sexual or drug use behavior or STI or HIV status.

Human subjects have the right to certain protections, including:

- The right to know that they are **participating** in a study.
- The right to know the **procedures** of the study.
- The right to know the possible **risks** involved in participating in the study.
- The right to know the possible **benefits** of participating in the study.

To help ensure privacy and confidentiality for evaluation participants, it is important to:

- Provide a private place for participants to complete evaluation surveys or interviews, out of the view or earshot of other clients or program staff. When many people must complete surveys in the same room, allow them to spread themselves out or turn their chairs. When this is not possible, give each participant a blank sheet of paper that they can use to cover their answers as they complete the survey.

- Assign an individual identification number to each evaluation participant for use on evaluation surveys or other data records. This is safer than using personal identifying information such as name, date of birth, or Social Security number. Keep the key that links identification numbers to names separate from the data.

- Keep all data and related information in locked cabinets. Allow access to these materials on a need-to-know basis only.

- In evaluation reports, never include participants' names or any other information that can uniquely identify them. For example, if your program had only one Native American participant, do not report findings separately for that person, because it will be easy for others to identify who he or she is.

**Figure 4-1  Tips: Protecting privacy and confidentiality.**

- The right to **refuse** participation in the study at any time.
- The right to have their **privacy** protected throughout the course of the study.

These protections apply to **all** research projects involving human subjects, including program evaluation research.

## Why Is Human Subjects Protection Important?

Over the years, there have been many examples of abuse of human subjects in research. For example, in the infamous Tuskegee Syphilis Study (1930–1972), the U.S. Public Health Service denied more than 400 African-American men treatment for syphilis so that researchers could observe the progression of the disease. The subjects did not know that a simple treatment for syphilis was being withheld from them, and that they were suffering physically as a result of the denial of treatment. Although the worst offenses against human subjects' rights have generally taken place in the course of biomedical research, human subjects involved in behavioral research can also suffer harm from their participation and are entitled to all of the same rights and protections as participants in biomedical studies.

## Key Terms for Human Subjects Protection

A number of key terms used in discussion of human subject protection issues have specific meanings within a research and evaluation context. Several of these terms and their definitions are summarized below.

*Privacy* refers to people's ability to keep their personal information (e.g., physical, behavioral, emotional, intellectual, political, demographic, etc.) to themselves and to determine whether, how, and with whom it will be shared. Human subjects' privacy is maintained when they or the evaluators prevent others from accessing this information, unless the individuals themselves choose to make it public. Some tips for ensuring subjects' privacy are provided in Figure 4–1.

*Anonymity* is a state in which a person's individual identity or personal identifying information is unknown to others and cannot be discovered. To protect human subjects who participate in a study under a condition of anonymity, evaluators should not collect any potentially uniquely identifying information, such as name or Social Security number.

*Confidentiality* is the keeping private of information that individuals provide under the condition that it not be disclosed without their permission. Evaluators must keep all personal data that they collect confidential by either stripping it of all potentially uniquely identifying information (e.g., name, Social Security number) or by keeping such information in a locked storage facility. Evaluation reports should never link or permit the linkage of data to any specific individual (see also Figure 4–1).

An *Institutional Review Board (IRB)* is group of individuals who review research protocols and approve only those projects that adequately protect the welfare of human subjects recruited to participate in the study. Federally funded evaluation projects involving human subjects require IRB review, as do most evaluation projects conducted by university affiliates and other governmental entities.

## Informed Consent

Evaluators must obtain all study participants' express permission, or *informed consent*, to take part in a study. This includes participation in evaluation activities such as focus groups; written, computer-based, or oral surveys; group or individual interviews; medical exams; case file reviews; and onsite observations. Audio or video recordings of participants should also be made *only* with their informed consent.

To obtain informed consent, evaluators must provide prospective participants with sufficient information, in language that they can understand, to enable them to decide whether or not to participate in a study. In particular, evaluators should explain the study completely, outline the potential benefits and drawbacks of participation, and inform the individual that participation is voluntary and may be discontinued at any time. A participant's informed consent is documented on an *Informed Consent Form.* Those individuals who do not wish to participate should not sign a consent form or be included in the study.

Informed consent honors and respects individuals' rights and choices regarding research participation. Documentation of the decision to participate also ensures funders that individuals understand and are participating in the study voluntarily.

It is important to be aware that when working with evaluation participants under the age of legal consent in your state (i.e., minors), you will usually need to obtain the voluntary agreement of both the minor and the minor's parent(s) or guardian(s). Such voluntary agreement is called "assent" for the minor and "consent" for the parent or guardian. Your work setting may have additional rules or regulations concerning the involvement of minors in evaluation research.

## Cultural Competence, Protecting Human Subjects, and Informed Consent

A culturally competent evaluation pays particular attention to participants' culturally specific needs with respect to informed consent and privacy. Some of your participants, for example, may not be English-speaking, or English may not be their primary language. They may also or alternatively have low literacy skills in English or their native language. It is important that you provide all documents in an appropriate language or an alternative format. For example, you can read the consent form to participants and then obtain informed consent orally with the assistance of a witness.

This book's Tools 4–2 to 4–8 can help you to develop informed consent materials in English and Spanish and implement appropriate informed consent procedures.

## Who Is Responsible for Human Subjects Protection?

The main responsibility for human subjects protection rests with the evaluation team. This includes the primary evaluator or researcher and any other staff involved in administering, collecting, storing, sending, or analyzing surveys or other data. When an IRB is involved in the project, it assists the team by reviewing and

The National Institutes of Health (NIH) offers an online training course entitled "Human Participant Protections Education for Research Teams." It provides a further introduction to human subjects research participation and to the steps involved in protecting the rights and welfare of study participants. The course is available free of charge to the public. Key personnel on NIH-funded research projects involving human subjects are required to take the course before the release of their funding.

See http://cme.cancer.gov/clinicaltrials/learning/humanparticipant-protections.asp for further information.

**Figure 4-2  Tip: Free online human subjects training.**

approving proposed procedures and instruments and helping to address any concerns that participants may raise.

A free online course on human subjects protection is made available by the National Institutes of Health (NIH). See Figure 4–2 for further details.

# DISTINGUISHING PROCESS EVALUATION FROM OUTCOME EVALUATION

Both process and outcome evaluations can help improve the quality and effectiveness of an HIV prevention program.

## What Is a Process Evaluation?

Because even the most carefully designed programs often differ in practice from what was planned, it is important to document how the program is actually delivered. A process evaluation serves this purpose by addressing the following questions:

- What HIV prevention services or activities has the program provided, in comparison to what was planned?
- Who has received these services, in comparison to the population that the services were intended for?
- What resources were used to deliver services, in comparison to the resources that were allocated?
- How satisfied are staff and participants with the services as delivered?

Answering these questions will help you to improve your program, track and manage your resources more effectively, and facilitate accountability to your funders and your community. A process evaluation will also help you determine whether or not you are ready for an outcome evaluation (i.e., an assessment of program effects, or how your program has changed its participants—see later). For example, if you are not delivering the services you planned or reaching the population you targeted, you are unlikely to be achieving positive effects and should therefore not waste resources on an outcome evaluation. Ideally, an outcome evaluation will be accompanied by a concurrent process evaluation, so that the process findings can help shed light on the outcomes. Specifically, if your outcome findings are positive, having process data will help you to share with others how you achieved these outcomes. This will help researchers, funders, and colleagues at other agencies to replicate your procedures and findings in other settings. By contrast, if some outcome findings are negative, having process data will help you understand whether it was your underlying program theory, or problems encountered during implementation of your program, that led to the negative results. This will suggest ways to improve the program. An example of process and outcome findings, and the conclusions to be drawn from them, is provided in Figure 4–3.

| **Process finding** |
|---|
| Because of staff's and participants' different language backgrounds, staff were unable to implement "active learning" role-playing activities with program participants. |

| **Outcome finding** |
|---|
| Participant ability to negotiate condom usage with sexual partners did not improve from pre-program to post-program. |

| **Conclusion** |
|---|
| Language barriers that prevent staff from implementing role-play activities need to be addressed. This will afford participants more opportunities to practice and improve condom negotiation skills. |

**Figure 4-3  Example: Using process and outcome findings.**

## What Is an Outcome Evaluation?

An *outcome evaluation* can help you assess if your HIV prevention program actually achieved the desired effects on your participants. Most outcome evaluations of HIV prevention programs focus on changing participants' HIV-related knowledge, attitudes, beliefs, skills, intentions, and behaviors. Some also include an assessment of changes in relevant health status outcomes, such as HIV or STI infection status.

An outcome evaluation can help address one or more of the following questions:

- Did the program make a difference in participants' knowledge, attitudes, beliefs, skills, intentions, behaviors, or health status?
- If so, for how long were these effects sustained?
- For whom and under what circumstances was the program most effective?
- Was the program, or some other circumstance, responsible for the observed effects?
- What aspects of the program were responsible for the observed effects?

The best way to determine if it is your program—and not some other factor—that is responsible for observed effects is to include a *comparison group* in your evaluation. A comparison group is another group of persons who are similar in as many respects as possible to your participants (i.e., your *treatment group* or *intervention group*), except that they have not taken part in your HIV prevention program.

## How Do I Decide Which Type of Evaluation Is Right for My Program?

In order to determine whether a process or outcome evaluation (or both) is right for your HIV prevention program, consider the following questions:

1. **What is it that I would like to know?** Identify the questions that you and your colleagues would like your evaluation to answer.
2. **What are the needs of my community?** Understand the needs of your community and consider what type of evaluation can demonstrate how your program is meeting these needs.
3. **What are the needs of my funder?** Consider your funder's evaluation requirements and how they can best be addressed.
4. **What are the relevant policy debates?** Consider what policies, if any, you would like to influence and what type of evaluation can provide you with relevant findings to influence decision makers.

5. **What resources are available for an evaluation?** Consider how much time and money would be needed for each evaluation type, versus the time and money actually available for evaluation. Also consider program staff's and participants' willingness to participate in an evaluation.

It is important to keep in mind that an outcome evaluation is generally far more expensive than a process evaluation. To avoid wasting resources, it is important to undertake outcome evaluation only when you are sure that your program and agency are ready for it. The assessment of outcome evaluation readiness is discussed in greater detail later in this section.

You should also remember that neither process nor outcome evaluation is inherently culturally competent. It takes an intentional and concerted effort to ensure that any evaluation, regardless of the type or scope, incorporates culturally competent principles and practices.

## CONDUCTING A CULTURALLY COMPETENT PROCESS EVALUATION

A culturally competent process evaluation assesses program delivery in ways that take the needs, concerns, ideas, and beliefs of program participants, staff, and the broader community into account. Its design and execution, including formulation of research questions, selection of data collection and analysis methodologies, and interpretation of findings, are all shaped by an awareness and incorporation of local cultural norms (Snowden, 2003).

### Questions That a Culturally Competent Process Evaluation Can Answer

A culturally competent process evaluation can answer a number of important questions about your HIV prevention program.

- What services were delivered, compared to those planned in your program model?
- Who received services, compared to whom you intended to reach in your program model?
- What resources were used to implement the program, compared to what you budgeted?
- How satisfied were staff and participants with the program? Do they feel that it appropriately addressed participant needs?
- To what extent did staff and management adhere to principles and practices of culturally competent program implementation?

The answers to these questions will help you to be accountable to your stakeholders and plan to how to improve your program.

### Process Evaluation Planning

A successful process evaluation requires careful planning. The key steps in this planning process are summarized briefly here.

1. **Identify evaluation questions**. Involve diverse stakeholders in this process, including program staff and community leaders. Choose the questions that are most important to stakeholders to answer, in relation to available resources. Be sure to consider what evaluation questions your funder(s) would like answered.

2. **Determine data collection needs and methods**. Process evaluation data can be collected in a variety of ways. You should choose the methods that are appropriate to your evaluation questions, program structure, and resources, as well as the cultural background of your participants. For example, a written client satisfaction survey would not be appropriate for a population with very low literacy skills, unless it is read aloud with accompanying visual aids. Focus groups may need to be conducted separately with men, women, and transgendered individuals if cultural factors make it difficult or inappropriate for persons of different genders to speak openly about HIV-related topics in each other's presence. Further details on these and other common evaluation data collection methods are provided in Table 4–1. Tool 4–9: Process Evaluation Data Collection Matrix can help to identify the types of data and data collection methods that would be most appropriate for your program.

3. **Develop data collection instruments**. Program staff will be responsible for recording much of the process data, such as client registration information (e.g., on gender, age, race/ethnicity, etc.); program attendance information; and service delivery information (e.g., number of sessions provided). They may also complete surveys on their own satisfaction with the program, and they may lead focus groups or conduct interviews with program participants to get feedback on their reactions to the program and suggestions for improvement. It is therefore important to obtain extensive staff input in developing the forms or focus group or interview questions that will be used to collect this data. This will help to ensure that the questions reflect and address staff concerns, that data collection burden will be minimized, and that staff compliance with reporting requirements will be high. The last row of Table 4–1 provides information on how *protocol analysis* can be used to pilot test data collection instruments.

    If program participants will be asked to provide feedback on the program through surveys, interviews, or focus groups, it is important to obtain their input to the development of the forms or questions as well. This will help ensure that the format and content of the questions are culturally appropriate and comprehensible, and that they address the range of issues that are of greatest concern to clients.

    Tools 4–10 to 4–13 provide some sample process evaluation forms that can be adapted for use by a range of HIV prevention programs. A Spanish version of a sample participant satisfaction survey is provided in Tool 4–13.

4. **Pilot data collection instruments and procedures and revise as needed**: Try out your data collection instruments (i.e., your forms or focus group or interview questions) and procedures with a small number of people who represent the group (i.e., staff or program participants, as appropriate) who will be using them. Ask for their feedback on the clarity and appropriateness of the instruments and procedures, and use their suggestions to finalize your data collection plans.

5. **Protect human subjects**: Be sure that your evaluation data collection and analysis procedures comply with all federal, state, and local laws and your agency's policies regarding human subjects protection. Where applicable, you should obtain approval for your activities from an IRB, which oversees human subjects procedures (see earlier in this section). It is particularly important to ensure that all data collection, storage, and reporting procedures protect participants' privacy.

6. **Train staff to collect data**: Train staff in how to collect complete and accurate information, record it in a timely manner, and protect the rights of human subjects. In the case of program implementation logs and attendance sheets, for example, it is important for staff to record information during or just following *every program session*. If staff wait until many sessions have passed to make note of who attended or what was delivered, the information they record is likely to be inaccurate.

Some Common Evaluation Data Collection Methods (based in part on Snowden, 2003)

| Method | Description | Main Uses | Resources Required |
|---|---|---|---|
| FOCUS GROUPS | ■ A group of 5–10 program clients or staff is asked to respond to a series of open-ended questions (i.e., questions that require more than a yes/no or multiple choice answer).<br>■ A trained facilitator poses the questions and moderates the discussion, with the goal of actively involving all participants.<br>■ The session may be recorded on audiotape (with participant permission), or handwritten or typed notes may be made by designated note-takers as comments are spoken.<br>■ The data are analyzed for key themes and illustrative individual experiences. It is important to remember that these experiences are not necessarily representative of those of the larger community of which the individuals are a part. | ■ Obtain input on evaluation objectives, methods, or instruments.<br>■ Assess staff or client satisfaction with program implementation.<br>■ Provide insight into program effects documented through outcome evaluation. | ■ Staff to develop the questions and recruit participants.<br>■ A quiet, private room with circular seating.<br>■ A set of visuals to facilitate posing the questions (e.g., slides, flip chart, etc.).<br>■ An experienced focus group facilitator.<br>■ A recording device or 1–2 note-takers.<br>■ Participant incentives (e.g., snacks, gift certificates, etc.).<br>■ Staff to review the notes or recordings to identify key themes. |
| SEMISTRUCTURED INTERVIEWS | ■ A small number of program clients or staff are interviewed individually, using a list of open-ended questions (i.e., questions that require more than a yes/no or multiple choice answer).<br>■ The interviewer encourages participants to provide detailed responses and examples.<br>■ Each interview may be recorded on audiotape (with participant permission), or handwritten by the interviewer.<br>■ The data are analyzed for key themes and illustrative individual experiences. It is important to remember that these experiences are not necessarily representative of those of the larger community of which the individuals are a part. | ■ Obtain input on evaluation objectives, methods, or instruments.<br>■ Assess staff or client satisfaction with program implementation.<br>■ Provide insight into program effects documented through outcome evaluation. | ■ Staff to develop the questions and recruit participants.<br>■ A quiet, private room.<br>■ An interviewer.<br>■ An audiorecording device or notepad.<br>■ Participant incentives (e.g., snacks, gift certificate, etc.).<br>■ Staff to review the notes or recordings to identify key themes. |
| STRUCTURED SURVEYS AND INTERVIEWS | ■ Program clients or staff are asked to respond to a series of mainly closed-ended (i.e., yes/no and multiple choice) questions.<br>■ All members of each group (e.g., program participants, comparison group, etc.) receive the same questions and answer options, so that responses can be quantitatively analyzed and directly compared across individuals and (if applicable) over time.<br>■ Structured surveys are especially appropriate for use with large numbers of people.<br>■ For groups with limited literacy skills, the questions may be asked in a face-to-face interview, or with the assistance of a computer program that includes audio and/or video capabilities. | ■ Obtain input on evaluation objectives, methods, or instruments.<br>■ Assess staff or client satisfaction with program implementation.<br>■ Assess program effects on factors such as knowledge, attitudes, intentions, skills, and behaviors. | ■ Staff to develop the questions, recruit participants, and administer the survey or interview.<br>■ Copies of the printed survey (or computers or interview staff to deliver the survey orally).<br>■ A quiet, private setting for administering surveys.<br>■ Participant incentives (e.g., snacks, gift certificate, etc.).<br>■ Staff to input and analyze the survey data. |

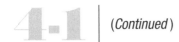   (*Continued*)

| Method | Description | Main Uses | Resources Required |
|---|---|---|---|
| PROTOCOL ANALYSIS | ■ Individuals or small groups review a survey instrument or set of interview questions in the presence of a researcher or evaluator and are encouraged to "think aloud" as they formulate a response to each question.<br>■ This personal reflection provides information on how the respondent understands the question and generates an answer.<br>■ A series of follow-up questions about the instrument may also be asked.<br>■ Responses may be recorded on audiotape (with participant permission), or handwritten by the researcher/evaluator. The data are analyzed for key issues that should be addressed in the further development of the instrument. | ■ Obtain input on evaluation instruments, such as question wording, appropriateness of instrument reading level, or overall instrument approach. | ■ Staff to plan what to ask participants to do, recruit participants, and work one-on-one or in small groups with participants.<br>■ Copies of the instrument to be reviewed.<br>■ A quiet, private room.<br>■ Participant incentives (e.g., snacks, gift certificate, etc.).<br>■ Staff to analyze the data for key issues or themes. |

Some additional tips for process evaluation planning and implementation are provided in Figure 4–4.

## Process Evaluation Data Analysis

Once the process data has been collected, you or an outside evaluator can conduct the analysis. Examples of types of analysis include:

■ *Comparing services delivered to services planned*—The content, delivery formats, and duration of planned program components, as defined in your program model (see Section 2), can be compared against the components as actually delivered, through an examination of your program implementation logs.

■ *Comparing population served to target population*—The number, gender, race/ethnicity, age, and other characteristics of the program's target population, as defined in your program model, can be compared to your actual program participants, using your registration and attendance logs.

■ *Comparing resources used against those allocated*—The program budget can be compared to your actual expenditures, per your accounting records.

- **Don't try to collect data on everything.** Among key stakeholders, decide on the most important evaluation questions and collect only the data that you need to address them.

- **Avoid duplication.** If you are already collecting process evaluation data to satisfy external funders' requirements, consider how you also might use this data for internal program purposes.

- **Review data as it comes in to be sure you are getting what you need.** If you find some key piece of information is missing, it may not be too late to revise data collection procedures and retrain staff so that you obtain the needed information.

**Figure 4-4 Tips for a better process evaluation.**

■ *Assessing staff and participant satisfaction*—Staff and participant satisfaction questionnaires may contain *closed-ended questions* (i.e., questions with a limited number of answer options, such as multiple choice questions) and *open-ended questions* (i.e., questions for which any number of answers is possible, such as fill-in-the-blank questions). Closed-ended questions can be analyzed quantitatively; for example, if program participants are asked to rate their satisfaction with the program materials on a scale of 1–5, then the average rating across participants can be calculated. Open-ended questions can be analyzed qualitatively; for example, what key themes emerge among responses to the question: "What was your favorite aspect of the program?" Focus group and interview transcripts or notes can be analyzed qualitatively for key themes as well.

■ *Assessing the cultural competence of program implementation*—Staff and participant satisfaction questionnaires, focus groups, and interviews can include questions about the cultural appropriateness of the program for the target population and community. Responses can be analyzed quantitatively or qualitatively, depending on the type of questions asked.

## USING PROCESS EVALUATION RESULTS

It is very important to work with key stakeholders (e.g., staff, program participants, and community leaders) to determine how to use your process evaluation findings to the benefit of your program, agency, and local community. There are many ways in which you can put your process evaluation to work to improve your program. For example, your results can:

■ Provide direction for program improvement by identifying barriers to achieving objectives and goals, and suggesting ways to overcome those barriers.
■ Inform decisions about the allocation of program resources.
■ Provide accountability to funders and the community.
■ Help enhance program and agency standing in the community.
■ Help you to secure new funding.
■ Help you to assess outcome evaluation readiness (see later in this section).
■ Shed light on outcome evaluation findings by suggesting where program delivery problems may be responsible for poor outcomes.
■ Point to ways in which programming is adhering to competent principles and practices and areas for improvement.

Once your process evaluation is complete, there are several important steps to follow that will help you translate your findings into meaningful program improvements.

1. **Share findings with key stakeholders**, such as program staff, community leaders, and program participants. Calling a meeting to present and discuss the results face to face can be particularly helpful.
2. **Develop a set of recommendations**, with stakeholder input, on how to address the findings.
3. **Identify and prioritize a list of action items for each recommendation**, also with stakeholder input. You may find it beneficial to brainstorm a list of potential actions first, and then narrow the list according to perceived community needs and available resources. The final list can be written up in a short action plan and circulated to key stakeholders for review.

# Using Evaluation Results to Improve an HIV and Substance Abuse Prevention Curriculum for Native American Youth

Researchers and Native American (and neighboring) communities in Northern Arizona were concerned about two complex, often related problems: HIV/AIDS prevention and the prevention of alcohol and other drug abuses (AOD). In response to these concerns, the Native American Prevention Project Against AIDS and Substance Abuse (NAPPASA) was formed. The organization set out to plan, implement, and evaluate youth-focused programs that linked both HIV and AOD prevention issues (Baldwin et al., 1996). Doing so in a culturally competent manner was an important goal.

NAPPASA developed all programs in partnership with local Native American organizations. Researchers, youth groups, and community members worked together to create a two-stage AOD and HIV prevention curriculum for eighth and ninth graders. The curriculum helps youth to build knowledge, social skills, and prevention skills around AOD and HIV risk behaviors. It also helps youth form and recognize new peer group norms around prevention, all in a manner consistent with Native American health beliefs and values.

During the early program planning stages, researchers conducted focus groups with youth and adults to better understand issues that shape AOD and HIV risks. For example, how did local youths communicate with each other—and with adults— about these issues? What norms, beliefs, and peer pressures were youth facing when it came to alcohol, substance abuse, and sexual risks? What barriers to prevention existed? The researchers learned that:

- Some youth were experiencing serious AOD troubles—including frequent impaired judgment and loss of consciousness—of which few adults were aware.
- Youth and adults differed in their ideas about the social meanings of AOD use, and even the types of places where AOD use occurs.

- Young males and females experienced communication challenges in discussing sexuality issues with each other, and with adults.
- There appeared to be links between heavy (illicit) substance use, binge drinking, and the increasing risk of HIV transmission among teens in rural communities.

Based on these findings, the researchers created a prototype prevention curriculum that was (a) responsive to youth perceptions and risk behaviors; and (b) addressed the consequences of AOD, especially as it related to HIV risk. The curriculum included:

- Individual and group exercises that helped participants with safer decision making, communication, and negotiation strategies when high or drunk.
- Biological, social, cultural, and psychological topics relevant to creating a Native American holistic approach to AOD and HIV prevention.
- Strategies for minimizing student embarrassment about these topics, including the use of two instructors (one male, one female) and sensitive cross-gender role playing about HIV and AOD risk reduction.

Next, the researchers set out to pilot test the prototype curriculum. Program participants completed a pre- and postintervention survey assessing their HIV and AOD prevention knowledge, attitudes, and risk behaviors. Postintervention, researchers conducted additional focus groups with students and instructors, as well as interviews with students and local advisory groups. Feedback indicated that the curriculum needed to (a) be more comprehensive; (b) be more visual and action-oriented, and (c) go further in reflecting traditional Native American health practices. In response, the curriculum was extended from 14 to 24 sessions to include additional topics, activities, teaching processes, and visual materials.

Local videos were produced, and existing videos were adapted. To increase the number of culturally relevant learning activities, an interactive student manual was added that complemented the logic and goals of the instructor manual.

The revised, culturally tailored curriculum was now ready to be implemented in nine schools. The researchers conducted process and outcome evaluations using student questionnaires, focus groups, and interviews with students, instructors, and advisors. Evaluation data were used to refine the curriculum even further and to better meet the needs of different age groups (i.e., eighth vs. ninth graders). This involved splitting the curriculum into two stages: one for eighth graders, and one for ninth graders that could either stand alone or build on skills and knowledge gained from participation in the eighth grade curriculum.

4. **Disseminate the process evaluation findings, recommendations and action plan to additional stakeholders**. You may wish to do this through a page on your Web site, an article in a newsletter, a formal report, or presentation at a meeting. Even if some of your findings are negative, disseminating them widely—along with a list of recommendations and corresponding action items—demonstrates your commitment to providing the best possible HIV prevention services. It also demonstrates to funders that you are taking action to use your resources as efficiently and effectively as possible.

It is also important to follow through on your action plan. As you do so, you should continue to collect and analyze process data from your program. This will permit you to assess whether the programmatic changes you have implemented are leading to improvements in service delivery. Tale 4–2 provides an example of how evaluation data were used to improve an HIV and substance abuse prevention curriculum for Native American youth.

## ASSESSING READINESS FOR CULTURALLY COMPETENT OUTCOME EVALUATION

Outcome evaluation constitutes the **best, most scientific way** to determine if your program is having the desired impact on your program participants' knowledge, attitudes, beliefs, skills, intentions, behaviors, or health status. Outcome evaluation can also provide information about how your program is producing the desired impact. This information is useful for documenting successes and challenges to funders, providing accountability to the local community, and increasing the efficiency and effectiveness of programming efforts. However, not every HIV prevention program is necessarily ready to conduct a culturally competent outcome evaluation. Before initiating outcome evaluation planning, it is important to assess agency and program readiness.

### Why Is It Important to Assess Outcome Evaluation Readiness?

It generally requires a significant investment of resources to:

- Decide on outcome evaluation research questions that reflect diverse stakeholders' interests.
- Develop methods and instruments that are appropriate for clients' circumstances and cultural backgrounds.
- Collect data from clients both before and after completion of program participation, without losing too many participants during the program or at follow-up data collection points.

■ Analyze and interpret the data in ways that are sensitive to client and community norms, values, and needs.

You should invest resources in an outcome evaluation only when you are likely to be able to complete these activities successfully and obtain useful findings.

## How to Assess Outcome Evaluation Readiness

The criteria listed here can help you to assess whether or not your program and agency are ready to conduct a culturally competent outcome evaluation.

1. **Strength of program design (Kirby, 2004; Sedivy, 2000).** You should have a clear understanding of what your program seeks to achieve (i.e., the goals and objectives) and how (i.e., the program components). Ideally, this information should be reflected in a *program model,* which is a chart or diagram that visually links program activities or services to desired changes in the target population. (For more on program models and the criteria for assessing their strength, see Section 2.) Your program design is not yet ready for an outcome evaluation if its design or program model: (1) lacks coherence or stakeholder consensus; (2) does not robustly incorporate and address local needs and assets, including cultural factors that influence HIV risk; or (3) is not based on known best practices in HIV prevention.
2. **Strength of program implementation (Sedivy, 2000).** A process evaluation can provide comprehensive data on service delivery strength. If you have not yet conducted a process evaluation, or if your findings show that you are not reaching the intended audience or delivering the intended content, or that staff or participants are dissatisfied with the program, then the program is unlikely to be ready for an outcome evaluation.
3. **Program participant and comparison group accessibility (Sedivy, 2000).** Most outcome evaluations depend on surveying or testing program participants both before and after they have participated in your HIV prevention intervention. You may also need to collect data from them several months or even a year or more after your program has ended to see if certain impacts persist or emerge. Because outcome evaluations ideally include a comparison group against which to measure changes in your intervention group (see later in this section), it is important to assess the availability of *both* your program participants and an appropriate comparison group for data collection over time before you decide to proceed with an outcome evaluation.
4. **Resource availability (Sedivy, 2000).** Outcome evaluations require a commitment of staff time and expertise, participant time, and financial and other resources. These burdens can vary considerably with evaluation design and the outcomes you would like to measure. It is important to carefully consider the availability of these resources and the burden an evaluation will place upon them when assessing outcome evaluation readiness.
5. **Ability to involve stakeholders**. To design and implement an outcome evaluation that reflects community values, beliefs, and needs, it is very important to involve community stakeholders in all outcome evaluation activities. If your agency does not have strong community ties and an ability to secure participation of community leaders and members in evaluation activities, you may not be ready to conduct a culturally competent outcome evaluation.

For help assessing your program against these criteria, see Tool 4–14: Outcome Evaluation Readiness Screening Checklist. By conducting such assessment, you can determine whether you are ready to conduct outcome evaluation.

# CONDUCTING A CULTURALLY COMPETENT OUTCOME EVALUATION

An outcome evaluation measures your HIV prevention program's effects or impacts. It involves collection and analysis of:

- *Pretest* or *baseline* data (i.e., data before the start of the program).
- *Posttest* or *postprogram* data (i.e., data collected at the end of the program and often at one or more follow-up points, such as 3, 6, or even 12 or more months later).
- Data describing the intervention, collected through a process evaluation.

An outcome evaluation can help you understand whether your program has achieved its goals and objectives, such as increasing program participants' HIV prevention-related knowledge and skills; changing their attitudes, beliefs, and behavioral intentions; decreasing their risk behaviors or increasing their protective behaviors; and decreasing STI or HIV infection rates. A set of questions that focus on the program's goals and objectives should guide an outcome evaluation.

A *culturally competent outcome evaluation* seeks to (a) understand the cultural norms, values, beliefs and practices of program participants and their communities, and (b) incorporate them into all evaluation activities, including identification of evaluation questions; development of a study design, methods, and instruments; and collection, analysis, and interpretation of the data (Hoban & Ward, 2003). When you are conducting a culturally competent outcome evaluation, it is important to avoid assumptions and stereotypes about program participants and their communities. It is also important to be aware that evaluation activities are not always neutral, but instead are based on ideas about how best to measure indicators and interpret observations. These ideas should be challenged and revised, as needed, based on knowledge of and input from program participants and community representatives.

## Outcome Evaluation Planning

Conducting a culturally competent outcome evaluation requires careful planning. Key planning steps and activities are summarized briefly here.

1. **Begin planning early**. It is best to begin planning for evaluation long before your program or program cycle begins. This will allow you to develop and pilot test data collection instruments prior to using them in the evaluation. It will also allow you to collect baseline data from participants before the program, so that you can measure changes in their knowledge, attitudes, behaviors, or other indicators over time. In addition, planning early will allow you to collect appropriate process data over the course of the program, so that information on the quality of service delivery can be used to help explain both positive and negative outcome findings.

2. **Identify what you want to measure.** Look at your program model or other program design documents to remind yourself of the program goals and objectives (i.e., desired changes in knowledge, attitudes, behaviors, skills, intentions, behaviors, or health status) that you had identified during program planning. Ask program stakeholders (e.g., staff, community leaders, and representatives of your target population) for their input on the goals and objectives to measure in outcome evaluation. Choose those that the group feels are most important and most feasible to measure, given the available resources.

   Keep in mind that the most rigorous measures of program success are HIV-related behaviors, such as those shown in Table 4–2, and health status indicators,

Examples of HIV Prevention-Related Behaviors (adapted from Card et al., 2001a)

| Behavior Type | Examples of Specific Behaviors |
|---|---|
| Sexual Behavior | ■ Postponement of sexual intercourse<br>■ Decreased frequency of sexual intercourse<br>■ Decreased number of sexual partners<br>■ Decreased frequency of sexual intercourse with partners who engage in high risk behaviors (e.g., injection drug use, prostitution, male-male sex)<br>■ Increased consistent use of effective condoms at every sexual contact<br>■ Substitution of lower risk sexual behaviors for high-risk sexual behaviors<br>■ Increased performance of other sex-related HIV prevention behaviors (e.g., increased condom purchasing and carrying) |
| Drug Injection Behavior | ■ Abstinence from injection drug use<br>■ Reduced frequency of injection drug use<br>■ Reduced sharing of needles and other drug-injection equipment/materials (e.g., cookers and filters)<br>■ Reduced reuse of needles<br>■ Increased disinfecting of needles (with bleach) |
| Prenatal Transmission Behavior | ■ Increased contraceptive use among HIV+ females |
| HIV/AIDS Treatment Behaviors* | ■ Increased adherence to prescribed antiretroviral therapy regimens (e.g., dosage amount, timing, etc.) |

* Adherence to treatment can reduce the body's viral load and in turn the risk of spreading HIV to others.

such as STI infection status and HIV serostatus. Think about including at least one or more behavioral measures in your evaluation.

3. **Choose measurement methods.** Once you have determined what to measure, think about how best to measure it. For example, you may decide to use a survey to measure changes in knowledge about HIV transmission, attitudes about condom use, and self-reports of sexual behavior. Further information on common evaluation data collection methods was provided previously in Table 4–1.

   It is important to keep in mind that no research method is inherently culturally competent. Therefore evaluation activities should be conducted in ways that reflect the norms, beliefs, and needs of your participants and community (Snowden, 2003). For example, surveys may need to be administered orally, with culturally appropriate visual aids, to clients with limited literacy.

4. **Design and pilot test measurement instruments**. Outcome evaluation instruments should use language, images, and examples that reflect the norms and practices of participants (Stanton et al., 1995). Once instruments are drafted, they should be pilot tested for clarity and appropriateness with representatives of the groups that will use them. One way to do this is to have a small number of people use each instrument and then provide feedback via a focus group.

   Table 4–1 provides additional information on how *protocol analysis* can be used to pilot test data collection instruments.

   Tools 4–15 and 4–16 provide sample English- and Spanish-language outcome evaluation surveys that may be adapted for use with different populations and programs. An example of how a culturally competent outcome evaluation instrument was developed for use with African-American youth is provided in Tale 4–3.

# 4-3    Developing a Culturally Competent Evaluation Instrument for an African-American AIDS Educational Intervention

Compared to other U.S. populations, African Americans have been disproportionately affected by the HIV/AIDS epidemic. Aware of this fact, Bonita Stanton and her colleagues at the Center for Minority Health Research at the University of Maryland were concerned about the lack of appropriate research instruments for assessing HIV risk behaviors among African Americans. Stanton and her colleagues decided to develop a new survey for monitoring the behavioral and health impact of an AIDS education program among urban, African-American pre- and early adolescents (Stanton et al., 1995).

In creating the survey, the team wanted to ensure it was both culturally relevant and age appropriate. They considered the following issues:

- How can we develop the survey and conduct the research in collaboration with the community where it will be used?
- How should we conceptualize the problem(s) the survey will address?
- What theoretical model of behavior change best applies to the survey?
- What language and delivery format should we use in the survey?

*Community collaboration.* The research team wanted to make sure they involved local youth in the design of the survey instrument. In focus groups, the researchers learned how local youth conceptualized the idea of "risk" and what they thought of various "protective" activities for reducing HIV risk. Focus group participants also offered their ideas on specific survey questions.

*Conceptualizing the problem(s).* The researchers wanted to make sure their survey instrument reflected concepts and practices that were meaningful to youth. For example, while adults might view the decision to initiate sex as directly related to decisions about condom use, local youth reported viewing these two processes as distinct, and using different factors to make the two decisions. Researchers used the youths' feedback to develop

four decision-making models or paradigms that reflected youths' actual decision-making processes. These models would be used in the study's evaluation component (see more on this later).

*Applying a model of behavior change.* Social/behavioral surveys should be developed using relevant theories of behavior change. The survey can then be used by researchers to examine the relationship between observed behaviors/behavior change and what the relevant theory says about them. (This strategy also helps researchers assess the appropriateness of the theory they have selected.) In developing their survey, Stanton and her colleagues utilized a social cognitive theory (see Section 2) called Protection Motivation Theory (PMT). This theory considers (a) how environmental and personal factors combine to become a threat, and (b) the various ways people adapt to these threats, using behaviors that are more or less successful.

The researchers used PMT concepts in focus groups to learn more about how youth thought about risk and protective behaviors. They also employed the youth decision-making models (noted earlier) to create evaluation questions for each PMT risk behavior area (e.g., using drugs, having unprotected sex, etc.) This helped researchers develop a series of specific questions regarding each distinct behavior (e.g., "Have you ever smoked marijuana?" "Have you ever sold marijuana?"), and to assess the relationship between youth behaviors and the PMT theory itself.

*Language and delivery format.* Surveys need to be presented using language and delivery formats that respondents can understand and respond to accurately. Word choice and even grammar can vary by ethnicity, age, and educational level, as can familiarity with different types of questions (e.g., true/false, multiple choice). Surveys also can be delivered in different formats (e.g. self-administered, interviewer-administered, using a paper survey versus an online survey) that affect people's comfort level when responding. This is especially true when the questions concern illegal or socially unacceptable activities, such as using drugs or having multiple sexual partners. To be effective in identifying behavior/behavior change, a survey instrument must take all of these factors into account. This can greatly enhance the *validity* of a survey instrument—the likelihood that the survey instrument will collect the type of information that it claims to be collecting.

Stanton and her team wanted to make sure that the survey they developed was comprehensible to the target audience and a suitable length. They pilot tested the survey in four waves with different youth, in different sites, using different formats. They also conducted *ethnographic research*, making observations of people taking the survey and interviewing community members firsthand to hear their survey recommendations.

The researchers' use of multiple methodologies yielded several important, concrete recommendations for survey refinement. These included:

- Shortening the survey from 2 hours to 60 minutes.
- Deleting questions that youth could not or would not answer honestly.
- Rethinking and rewording questions to make sure they reflected the distinctions youth made between related behaviors (initiating sex vs. condom use; selling drugs vs. using drugs).
- Administering the survey through a computer with audio capability, rather than in written format or with an in-person facilitator.

The team incorporated these changes into the final instrument, which was then retested and validated with different groups of respondents. By culturally tailoring the survey instrument in these ways, the researchers were able to collect highly valid data on the *specific* sex- and drug-related attitudes and behaviors that were putting the target audience at particular risk of HIV infection.

5. **Decide whether to include a comparison group.** A comparison group is a group that is as similar as possible to your program participants with respect to demographic, cultural, and HIV risk factors, but that does not experience the same intervention during the evaluation period. They may receive no intervention or an alternate intervention. The function of the comparison group is to help you determine whether or not it is your program (rather than some other factor) that is having an impact on program participants. When an outcome evaluation includes random assignment of evaluation study participants to treatment and comparison groups, the comparison group is called a *control group.* Including a control group is considered a "gold standard" in outcome evaluation. This means it is considered to be the most scientifically accurate way to measure the effectiveness of a program. However, it is not always easy or appropriate to create a control group because of legal, ethical, or logistical considerations. For example, it may be unethical or even illegal to deny or delay access to your HIV prevention service to anyone who is eligible to participate.

   Including a comparison group (of any type) in an evaluation study can be costly, as it is generally necessary to collect the same data from both program participants and the comparison group, according to the same schedule (i.e., at pretest and one or more posttest points), to ensure that the two groups can be compared accurately. In considering whether or not to include a comparison group in your evaluation, it is important to weigh the potential costs and benefits of the various options.

6. **Set up a mechanism for linking subjects to data.** Most outcome evaluation data collection procedures should include a means of linking individual treatment and comparison group members to their data. This will allow you to measure change in study participants by analyzing data from only those who complete both a pre- and a posttest. Such linkage will also allow you to examine how program attendance level affects outcomes.

To help with data linkage, it is a good idea to assign each participant a unique number that is created solely for the purposes of the evaluation (rather than using an existing personal identifier, such as name, date of birth, Social Security number, etc). This number should appear on each data source that pertains to the participant (e.g., pretest, posttest, attendance information). A separate key that links the study identification number to the subject's name should be stored in a locked cabinet apart from the data.

It should be noted that a data collection procedure that uses this kind of linkage system cannot be considered anonymous, because there is a way for the evaluators to link the data to individual participants. However, as long as the participants' identities are not disclosed beyond the immediate evaluation team, the survey can be considered confidential.

7. **Determine data collection periodicity.** An outcome evaluation should collect data at multiple points over time to determine a program's impacts. As a part of the outcome evaluation planning process, it is important to decide when, in addition to baseline, you will collect data. Most outcome evaluations collect data at baseline and immediately upon program conclusion, to assess short-term program effects. You may want to consider collecting data from clients at additional points—such as 3, 6, 12, or more months after program participation—in order to assess intermediate and long-term program effects. The key is to define data collection points that reflect when you could reasonably expect to see changes in the principal outcome indicators. For example, if you are working with young teens, most of whom have not yet become sexually active, you may not be able to measure differences in sexual behavior between program and comparison groups until a year or more after program completion.

In most cases, data should be collected from program and comparison groups at the same time, to help ensure that any differences between the two groups are the result of the intervention, and not external factors such as participants' maturation or changes in community-wide norms, infrastructure, or other services. However, if the intervention being evaluated is short (e.g., one or two sessions held over a day or a week), and your comparison group does not participate in a alternate intervention at the same time, then it is reasonable for data collection practices to diverge somewhat across the groups. Specifically, you can collect baseline, immediate posttest, and follow-up data from your program group, but only collect baseline and follow-up data from your comparison group. This is because your comparison group will not be expected to change in the very short time period (i.e., a day or a week) between the pretest and the intervention group's immediate posttest.

8. **Plan for study attrition (dropout).** It is likely that some participants will not complete the program or will not be reachable at the data collection follow-up points. They may drop out as a result of lack of interest or schedule conflicts, move away from the area, or have to discontinue participation for other reasons. The loss of participants during a program or study is referred to as *attrition*. High rates of attrition can threaten the validity of a study because the findings for just a small subset of the original participants do not necessarily represent what would be found for the group as a whole. Attrition can also make the number of study participants so low that it is difficult to perform statistical tests on the data that can establish whether the program really made a difference.

It is therefore important to take steps during the evaluation planning period to prevent or reduce attrition. For example, you can set aside funds (or get donations) for appropriate incentives, such as payments, gift cards, T-shirts, condoms, or food, to help maintain high participation rates at program sessions and follow-up data collection activities. Members of the program's target population should be asked for input on what types of incentives would be most appropriate and useful. In addition, you may want to plan to include a larger number of participants in your study at the beginning than you might need to measure the outcome you are investigating. If some drop out, you may still have a large enough number to track program impact in a meaningful way.

9. **Ensure protection of human subjects.** As you collect, analyze, interpret, and report on the data, it is essential to ensure study participants' privacy and safety. Putting human subjects safeguards in place during the evaluation planning period helps ensure that confidentiality will be maintained and that participants' rights will be respected. Be sure that your evaluation design and methods comply with all applicable laws and regulations regarding human subjects protection. For examples:

   ■ Where applicable, you should obtain approval from an IRB, which oversees human subjects procedures (see earlier in this section, in the discussion on protecting human subjects).

   ■ You should plan to secure informed consent from participants (and parental consent and youth assent from any minors who participate).

   ■ You should ensure that all data collection, storage, analysis, and reporting procedures keep the identity of study participants and their individual responses private. For example, as indicated above, you should keep all data separate from any key that links the data to individuals. Store all of this information in a locked, secure place to which only authorized personnel have access.

10. **Train staff to collect the data (if applicable).** If the data will be collected by program staff (as opposed to an outside evaluation team), it is important to train them in the data collection procedures, including relevant issues concerning protection of human subjects. This will help ensure that the evaluation proceeds smoothly and that the data are complete and of high quality.

## Data Collection, Analysis, and Interpretation

It is important to collect data from evaluation participants according to the schedule established during the evaluation planning period. Data collection processes should be monitored to ensure that the right data are being collected at the right time, according to the agreed-on procedures, and that human subjects are being appropriately protected.

The data should be organized and analyzed using techniques that are appropriate to the evaluation design and methods. (Tool 4–17: Software and Online Tools provides a list of some software packages and free online tools that are commonly used to organize and analyze outcome evaluation data.) You may want to ask an appropriate external evaluator (see later in this section) to help you with these processes if you do not have a staff member who is knowledgeable about data analysis methods and tools that would be appropriate for your study.

Once the data have been organized and analyzed, you will have a set of findings that reveal whether or not any significant changes have occurred in your participants, with respect to the indicators that you measured (e.g., knowledge, attitudes, behaviors, etc.). The data from a comparison group will help you determine if changes you observe are a result of your intervention, in particular, as opposed to one or more outside factors. It is important to involve representatives of your target population in interpreting the outcome findings, as they can likely offer perspectives and insights that differ from those of program staff or outside evaluators.

An example of a culturally competent outcome evaluation process is provided in Tale 4–4, which describes the evaluation of an HIV prevention program for Spanish-speaking migrant farm workers. Tale 4–5 reminds us of the importance of culturally competent outcome evaluation for advancing HIV prevention-related goals across diverse communities.

## 4-4    Culturally Competent Evaluation of an HIV Prevention Program for Latino Farm Workers

*Tres Hombres Sin Fronteras (Three Men Without Borders)* is an educational *fotonovela*—a pictorial/comic book—created as part of a program to educate Latino farm workers about the threat of HIV/AIDS (Conner, 2004). Designed by Ross Conner and his colleagues at the Center for Community Health Research at the University of California Irvine, *Tres Hombres* tells the story of three Mexican farm workers in the United States who meet sex workers in a migrant labor camp. One of the sex workers, Karla, functions as the story's educator, explaining the danger of unprotected sex and advocating condom use.

Before conducting a formal outcome evaluation of the program, the team decided to conduct a *formative evaluation*—an evaluation that takes place in the early stages of a program to revise and strengthen its activities. Staff at local community health clinics helped the researchers identify migrant farm workers who could review and provide feedback on the *fotonovela*, as well as on the evaluation design and instruments.

The farm workers provided crucial feedback on the structure and content of the program. In particular:

- They recommended that the character *Karla* serve as the HIV prevention educator in the story, because she is portrayed as a "high-class" sex worker whose business is sexual contact, and as someone who would have credibility with farm workers.
- They felt the structure of the story was valid and should not be changed. In the story, one of the three farm workers, Marco, serves as the point of identification for readers as the "good" example. He follows Karla's condom usage recommendation and does not contract HIV. A second farm worker, Sergio, serves as the "bad" example. He has sex with Lucy, another sex worker who does not use condoms. Lucy contracts HIV and infects Sergio, who then transmits HIV to his wife and unborn child.

- Finally, the farm workers felt that additional information was needed about where to obtain and how to use condoms. With farm workers as advisors, the research team produced a supplemental brochure entitled "Marco Aprende Cómo Protegerse" ("Marco Leans How to Protect Himself"). The brochure included several condoms inside, and was distributed with the original *fotonovela*.

The researchers also sought early feedback from the farm workers on how to best conduct an outcome evaluation survey among this population of predominantly Spanish-only speakers from rural Mexico. The survey would need to assess participants' HIV/AIDS related knowledge, attitudes, and behaviors. It would have to be administered to program participants before the program began, and one month after the program ended. The farm workers provided useful feedback that helped the research team understand the importance of:

- Conducting the evaluation using a small group format.
- Using oral-and-written survey administration formats (verbal directions accompanied by a set of written questions and multiple choice answers in Spanish).
- Replicating all questions and answers on a flipchart that a native speaker/facilitator would read, with his/her hand on the corresponding words on the flipchart as s/he spoke
- Using visual icons for survey questions and answer categories; this would help participants who did not read understand the questions and answers by matching the icons on the flipchart sheet with those on the written survey
- Beginning the survey with nonsensitive demographic questions first, to build rapport, then progressing to more sensitive questions on sexual behavior.

Overall, the researchers received very useful early feedback from the farm workers that helped (a) inform the intervention program's content, increasing the odds that the program would be effective; and (b) improve the researchers' outcome evaluation strategies, increasing the likelihood that the evaluation would capture these effects.

After the program materials and evaluation procedures were revised, the program was implemented with 10 matched camps of farm workers. The camps were paired based on similarity, with one randomly selected to receive the program initially, whereas the other served as the comparison group and did not receive the program until a month later. The evaluation showed positive program effects, with those in the treatment camp showing small but significant changes in sexual health knowledge, significant changes in attitudes, and improvements in condom usage.

## 4-5 Evaluating Community-Based HIV Prevention Programs for Asian and Pacific Islander Americans

Frank Wong and his colleagues from the Fenway Community Health Center in Boston noticed a lack of published reports about AIDS service organizations targeting Asian and Pacific Islander (API) Americans. Together with colleagues from the University of North Texas, they decided to review and profile six community-based API HIV prevention programs. They paid particular attention to programs that focused on men who have sex with men (MSM) (Wong et al., 1998).

The team sought to understand and describe how the six programs functioned in terms of (1) prevention and services, (2) research and evaluation, and (3) advocacy and policy. The six programs they selected represented the U.S. sites with the largest percentages of APIs, as well as subgroups within the API population with the largest percentages of adult AIDS cases. All six programs had an API and HIV prevention focus; some offered services to HIV-positive clients as well. The programs included:

■ a health center in Honolulu
■ a wellness center in San Francisco
■ an intervention team in Los Angeles
■ a New York City API coalition
■ a Philadelphia AIDS services program
■ a Massachusetts prevention project

Using data from telephone interviews with key program staff, the research team produced an historical and organizational profile of each program. The profiles included a review of each program's mission, services, and evaluation activities. Some highlights from their research are as follows:

*Agency histories*: The programs had not been in existence for very long; three (of six) were less than 6 years old and three had been running for a little over a decade. Five of the six programs had originated from gay or bisexual communities.

*Target populations*: The programs were aimed at diverse audiences, including API gay men, pregnant women and families, pregnant and parenting teens, bisexuals, lesbians, injection drug users, commercial sex workers, heterosexuals, MSM, youth, and transgender groups, among others.

*Services*: The six organizations offered a range of HIV-related services, including one-on-one outreach; distribution of printed educational materials; HIV testing and counseling; case management; and interpretation and translation services.

Only two organizations offered a telephone hotline, likely because of the difficulty and expense of providing language-appropriate services to the many diverse API groups. Nonetheless, all programs delivered HIV services in a number of major API languages, as well as English. Some of the organizations also offered additional services suited to the specific needs of their clients. These included Internet services for queer youth, a prevention case management "village" project to build a sense of community among at-risk API MSM, and paid, on-call bilingual peer advocates.

*Evaluation efforts*: All six programs had conducted internal process evaluations to assess their activities and services; one was also using an external evaluator required by the program funder. However, at the time of the data collection, no outcome evaluations had been conducted by any of the programs.

Overall, the researchers found that existing HIV prevention programs for API groups had made significant achievements in their communities. They were not only addressing risk factors for HIV infection, but also supporting community-wide processes that contributed to community strength and unity. However, ongoing needs and challenges remained. For example, there was still a lack of:

- Knowledge among API ethnic groups about the symptoms of HIV/AIDS and how the virus is spread.
- Comprehensive, research-based HIV prevention programs that were culturally tailored for APIs.

- Systematic evaluation data demonstrating the short-term outcomes and long-term impact of HIV programs targeting API groups.

The team concluded that more work is needed to further reduce the spread of HIV and to increase public health awareness among diverse API communities. They proposed both short-term and long-term objectives for meeting these goals:

*Short term*: More data is needed to shed light on how HIV affects API groups. Future research should focus on collecting data on HIV seroprevalence rates, HIV-related risk behavior, and knowledge, attitudes, and beliefs related to HIV risk in API communities. The data should be used to develop additional HIV prevention activities and services appropriate for API communities.

*Long term*: Data collected from evaluations of HIV prevention programs should be used to develop more comprehensive strategies to fight HIV in API communities. In particular, HIV prevention needs to be understood as part of a holistic approach to health, one that promotes culturally competent care overall. Future strategies should also focus on how to integrate HIV prevention into other health prevention activities for APIs. For example, if HIV testing is made part of family planning and adolescent health programming, it is less likely to be stigmatized and resisted.

## Using Outside Evaluators

As was indicated earlier, depending on the types of questions you would like an outcome evaluation to answer, the data that will need to be collected, and the analyses that will need to be performed, you might consider hiring an *outside* (or *external*) *evaluator* to help with one or more aspects of the evaluation. Specifically, a professional evaluator can assist with evaluation design, instrument development, data management (e.g., organization, coding, entry into a computer, cleaning), data analysis, and report writing. The following steps can help you to select an outside evaluator who is a good match for your needs:

1. Decide on specific evaluation questions and the resources available to measure them, and share this information with potential evaluators.
2. Review candidate evaluators' sample reports and references.
3. Consider candidate evaluators' experience working with HIV prevention programs and working with your target population or similar cultural groups.
4. Review candidate evaluators' proposed evaluation designs, methods, and timelines.
5. Clarify what each candidate evaluator would require of your staff and participants.
6. Decide whether you want results to be made public, even if unfavorable.

7. Once you select an evaluator, determine roles, responsibilities, deliverables, and costs ahead of time, and put them in writing.

# REPORTING OUTCOME EVALUATION FINDINGS

Reporting on your outcome evaluation findings can demonstrate your commitment to using your HIV prevention resources as effectively as possible. It can also open up more opportunities for dialogue with stakeholders about the best ways to address the culturally specific prevention needs of your program participants and community. However, it is important to be aware of how your findings—particularly negative findings—may have an adverse impact on already marginalized communities. For this reason, you should work with program staff and community leaders to determine how best to report findings to external parties, such as funders, policy makers, and the general public.

The following steps can help you to decide how to share what you have learned about your program:

1. **Identify your audiences**. Different groups are interested in knowing what you have learned and how you propose to respond to evaluation findings. But what and how much they want to know will vary. For example, funders may want to know far more about your data analysis methods than community members will. Decide who your key audiences are and how much information should be provided to each.
2. **Choose an appropriate medium and format.** Because of the differences in audiences discussed above, your findings (and any corresponding recommendations and action items) should be made available in different mediums and formats. For example, you may wish to disseminate information through a page on your website, an article in a newsletter, a formal report, or presentation at a meeting. The format of the findings should also be tailored to the audience—for example:
   - A short written summary that focuses mainly on key changes in knowledge, behaviors, opinions, or attitudes for community members.
   - A longer report research design and data analysis methods for funders. (See Figure 4–5 for an overview of a typical evaluation report format.)
   - A brief PowerPoint presentation of key evaluation methods and findings for agency Board Members.

---

An evaluation report typically has the following sections. You can place greater or lesser emphasis on particular sections, according to your audience. You also can adapt this format for use in an oral presentation to an agency Board of Directors or funder.

1. **Summary**: Includes an overview of the program, the evaluation questions and methods, and the evaluation findings.

2. **Program Background**: Reviews community needs and assets, the program's target population, and the program's goals, objectives, components, and staffing.

3. **Evaluation Description**: Describes the evaluation questions and the evaluation design and methods and their limitations.

4. **Study Results**: Presents specific findings in summary tables, graphs, or lists. Explains major points revealed by the data.

5. **Discussion**: Interprets the findings, including explanations or insights about what occurred and why.

6. **Conclusions and Recommendations**: Restates key findings. Lists recommendations appropriate to findings, and proposed action items (if determined).

**Figure 4-5  Tip: Organization of an evaluation report.**

Tool 4–18: Matrix for Disseminating Your Findings can help you to identify the various audiences and dissemination formats for your findings.

3. **Link positive findings to community needs.** Most audiences will want to know if your program was successful in addressing community needs. Link positive outcome evaluation findings to specific community problems or concerns, as identified in the needs and assets assessment work (see Section 2) or earlier evaluation studies that led to the development or refinement of your program.

4. **Present and explain negative findings.** Presenting your findings honestly, even if they are negative, can provide an opportunity to identify reasons for the findings, and build trust in the community. They also give program staff, community members, and funders the opportunity to address these weaknesses proactively, prior to the next program cycle. It is important to remember that few programs ever achieve everything they set out to achieve.

5. **Consider the impact on community empowerment.** Evaluation findings—both positive and negative—can sometimes be used in ways that you did not expect or intend. For example, someone might use them to reinforce problematic, inaccurate, or stereotypical views of particular cultural groups, even when there is no actual basis for this in your results. Be sure to present your findings in a manner that is sensitive to individual, community, and cultural group concerns and that can empower the individuals and groups you seek to serve (King et al., 2004).

6. **Connect findings to action.** Reporting evaluation findings offers an important opportunity to build community support for future action. Positive results can be leveraged to garner additional funding and community support, as well as to expand program scope and services. Negative findings can provide a foundation for specific programmatic changes to increase cultural competence, efficiency, and effectiveness. Connect your findings to recommendations and proposed action steps. Solicit feedback from a broad range of stakeholders through a focus group, community meeting, or other group format. Incorporate their suggestions into concrete action steps, some of which you can implement in the short term and others that you can work toward in the future.

## USING OUTCOME EVALUATION FINDINGS

Once you have conducted an outcome evaluation, it is important to translate what you have learned into a plan for action that will benefit your programming efforts. As discussed earlier, a key first step is to share your findings with program staff and community leaders. Together, you can form an advisory board or committee that develops a set of recommendations. These recommendations may concern:

- Changes to program content, formats, timing, or staffing, so that the program is more effective in recruiting and retaining participants and achieving its short-term objectives and long-term goals.
- Changes to evaluation methods or procedures, so that they are more cost-effective.
- Strategies for sustaining the program through new funding sources or increased volunteer support.
- Plans to disseminate information about the program to other agencies and/or to replicate the program in new sites.

You may find it beneficial to brainstorm a list of potential actions first, and then to narrow the list according to perceived community needs and available resources. Developing a timeline and assigning roles and responsibilities for specific actions can help ensure that the plan will be implemented.

It is also important to follow through on your action plan. As you do so, you should continue to evaluate your program. This will permit you to assess whether the changes or new strategies you have implemented are achieving the intended goals.

## REFERENCES

Baldwin, J., Rolf, J. E., Johnson, J., Bowers, J., Benally, C., & Trotter, R. T. (1996). Developing culturally sensitive HIV/AIDS and substance abuse prevention curricula for Native American youth. *Journal of School Health, 66*(9), 322–327.

Brach, C., & Fraser, I. (2000). Can cultural competency reduce racial and ethnic health disparities? A review and conceptual model. *Medical Care Research and Review, 57*(1), 181–217.

Butterfoss, F. D., Goodman, R. M., & Wandersman, A. (1996). Community coalitions for prevention and health promotion: Factors predicting satisfaction, participation, and planning. *Health Education Quarterly, 23*(1), 65–79.

Card, J. J., Benner, T., Shields, J. P., & Feinstein, N. (2001a). The HIV/AIDS Prevention Program Archive (HAPPA): A collection of promising prevention programs in a box. *AIDS Education and Prevention, 13*(1), 1–28. Retrieved September 14, 2005, from http://www.socio.com/progarticle.pdf

Card, J. J., Brindis, C., Peterson, J. L., & Niego, S. (2001b). *Guidebook: Evaluating teen pregnancy prevention programs* (2nd ed.). Los Altos, CA: Sociometrics Corporation.

Conner, R. F. (2004). Developing and implementing culturally competent evaluation: A discussion of multicultural validity in two HIV prevention programs for Latinos. *New Directions for Evaluation, 102* (Summer), 51–65.

The Florida Department of Health. (2004). Community health status and improvement planning terminology. Retrieved August 1, 2005, from http://www.doh.state.fl.us/planning_eval/CHAI/Resources/FieldGuide/6CommHealthStatus/CHSATerminology.htm

Fortier, J. P., Convissor, R., & Pacheco, G. (1999). *Assuring cultural competence in health care: Recommendations for national standards and an outcomes-focused research agenda.* Washington, DC: Department of Health and Human Services and Resources for Cross Cultural Health Care.

Hoban, M. T., & Ward, R. L. (2003). Building culturally competent college health programs. *Journal of American College Health, 52*(3), 137–141.

King, J. A., Nielsen, J. E., & Colby, J. (2004) Lessons for culturally competent evaluation from the study of a multicultural initiative. *New Directions for Evaluation, 102*(Summer), 67–80.

Kirby, D. (2004). *BDI logic models: A useful tool for designing, strengthening, and evaluating programs to reduce adolescent sexual risk-taking, pregnancy, HIV, and other STDs.* Retrieved July 3, 2005, from http://www.etr.org/recapp/BDILOGICMODEL20030924.pdf

LaFrance, J. (2004). Culturally competent evaluation in Indian Country. *New Directions for Evaluation, 102* (Summer), 39–50.

Miller, R. L. (2003). Adapting an evidence-based intervention: Tales of the Hustler Project. *AIDS Education and Prevention, 15*(Suppl A), 127–138.

Office for Human Research Protections, U.S. Department of Health and Human Services (HHS). (2005). Institutional review board guidebook glossary. Retrieved September 19, 2005, from http://www.hhs.gov/ohrp/irb/irb_glossary.htm

Sedivy, V. (2000). *Evaluation readiness assessment guide: Is your program ready to evaluate its effectiveness?* Los Altos, CA: Sociometrics Corporation.

Snowden, L. (2003). *Toward culturally competent evaluation in health and mental health.* Woodland Hills, CA: The California Endowment. Retrieved January 16, 2005, from http://www.calendow. org/evaluation/pdf/TowardBook.pdf

Stanton, B., Black, M., Feigelman, S., Ricardo, I., Galbraith, J., Li, X., et al. (1995). Development of a culturally, theoretically and developmentally based survey instrument for assessing risk behaviors among African-American early adolescents living in urban low-income neighborhoods. *AIDS Education and Prevention, 7*(2), 160–177.

Wong, F. Y., Chng, C. L., & Lo, W. (1998). A profile of six community-based HIV prevention programs targeting Asian and Pacific Islander Americans. *AIDS Education and Prevention, 10*(Suppl A), 61–76.

## Tool 4-1 Who Can Help You Carry Out a Culturally Competent Evaluation?[1]

Working with community leaders and other stakeholders will contribute to the design and execution of a culturally competent program evaluation. The table below can help you identify parties inside and outside your agency who might participate in your evaluation. Be sure to think broadly—for example, you may wish to include the names of organizations that might help your evaluation by donating materials or services, such as incentives for evaluation participants, data analysis software, or volunteer time. In the far right column, be sure to specify the kind of assistance that each party might provide.

To fill in the table below on your computer (using the file on the CD-ROM), click on the gray-shaded area in the box you would like to type in. (Note that the gray shading will not appear in printouts of this document.) Alternately, you may photocopy this tool (for your use only) and complete it by hand or typewriter.

| Name of Individual or Organization | Address, Phone, Fax, E-Mail | Interest or Expertise | Possible Evaluation Task |
|---|---|---|---|
|  |  |  |  |
|  |  |  |  |
|  |  |  |  |
|  |  |  |  |
|  |  |  |  |
|  |  |  |  |
|  |  |  |  |
|  |  |  |  |

[1] Adapted from Card, J. J., Brindis, C., Peterson, J. L., & Niego, S. (2001). *Guidebook: Evaluating teen pregnancy prevention programs* (2nd ed., Exercise 4.1). Los Altos, CA: Sociometrics Corporation.

# Tool 4-2 Explaining Human Subject's Rights and Informed Consent: Sample Script

Program staff members can utilize—or modify as needed—the following script to explain human subjects' rights and informed consent procedures to participants. Remember that it is necessary to inform all participants that an evaluation will take place and what it will entail, as well as afford them the opportunity to choose not to participate. **This script is not intended to address all of the issues that may need to be raised concerning human subjects' rights and informed consent, but it can serve as a helpful starting point.**

## A. BEFORE YOU DISTRIBUTE CONSENT FORMS:

(Note: See Tools 4–4 and 4–5 for sample *written* consent forms in English and Spanish, respectively; see Tools 4–7 and 4–8 for sample *oral* consent forms in English and Spanish, respectively.)

*"We would like to ask you to participate in a research study that is designed to evaluate the effectiveness of <program name>. Participating in the evaluation will involve <**explain evaluation activities that the person is being asked to engage in, such as completing a survey at intervals x, y, and z that will ask questions about HIV/AIDS-related knowledge or drug use and sexual behaviors**>. Your answers to these questions will be kept confidential, meaning that your name will never be linked to your answers in any reports or articles."*

*"We would appreciate your participation in this study. With your help, we can learn how to better serve our community. Your participation in this study is completely voluntary. You may refuse to participate in this study now, or at any time in the future. If you choose not to participate in this evaluation, you can still participate in this program and in other programs at our agency that you would otherwise be eligible to attend."*

*"If you choose to participate in this evaluation study, you have certain rights:*

- *You have the right to know you are participating in a study.*
- *You have the right to know the risks and benefits of participating in this study.*
- *You have the right to withdraw from the study now, or at any other time, without penalty*
- *You have the right to have your privacy protected throughout the study."*

*<**IF APPLICABLE:**> "This study has been approved by an Institutional Review Board (IRB), which is responsible for ensuring that your rights are protected. If, at any time, you are concerned with the manner in which this research is being undertaken, you may contact a member of the IRB. The contact information is on the informed consent form that I am about to give you." <**If participants are not literate and the consent form is to be read to them, substitute "read to you".**>*

## B. AFTER YOU DISTRIBUTE CONSENT FORMS:

*"This form is used to provide you with information regarding the evaluation study. Please read this document carefully. <**If participants are not literate and the consent form is to be read to them, substitute "please listen carefully as I read this document to you."**> It outlines what will be requested of you and what you will gain from participating. If you have any questions, please feel free to ask me."*

*<**Allow time for potential participants to read the forms. If the forms were read to them, give them a few moments to think about the information they just received.**>*

*"If you would like to participate in our evaluation study, please sign and date the form. One copy of the form is yours to keep, the other copy needs to be handed back to me." <**Modifications may be needed for persons who are not able to sign their name.**>*

# Tool 4-3 Written Informed Consent Checklist

The checklist below can help you to take the steps necessary to obtain written informed consent from evaluation participants. Place an "x" in the square box (☐) as you complete each item on the list. (To do this on your computer—using the file on the CD-ROM—use your cursor to click on the box. To remove an "x" from a box, click on the box again.)

☐ 1. Develop your Informed Consent Form. *(See Tools 4–4 to 4–5 for templates.)*

☐ 2. *(If applicable:)* Obtain Institutional Review Board (IRB) approval for your Informed Consent Form and procedures involving human subjects.

☐ 3. Review your Informed Consent Form.
  ☐ Make sure you are familiar with the content of the form so you can readily answer any participant questions.

☐ 4. Describe the Informed Consent Form to participants.
  ☐ Explain to all potential evaluation participants (including members of treatment and comparison groups) what informed consent is and why they need to sign the form if they choose to participate.

☐ 5. Answer participant questions, if any.

☐ 6. Distribute consent forms to all study participants.
  ☐ Ensure that each participant receives **two** copies of the consent form.

☐ 7. Ensure proper form completion.
  ☐ Make sure participants read the form completely.
  ☐ Those who are willing to participate must sign and date the form.

☐ 8. Collect one signed copy from each participant; keep it on file in a secure location.

☐ 9. Ensure that each participant keeps the second copy of the consent form.

☐ 10. Document which participants signed and returned the form.
  ☐ Retain a list of those participants who have completed the form. At each data collection point, you will need to use the list in order to identify who should participate in the ongoing evaluation.
  ☐ Remember to safeguard the privacy of these names by keeping them in a locked, limited-access storage facility.

**NOTE:** Remember that if your evaluation will involve persons under the legal age of consent (i.e., age 18 in most U.S. states), you must usually get *both* consent from the parent or guardian and assent from the minor for the minor to participate.

# Tool 4-4 Sample Informed Consent Template (English)

The template below can be used to develop an English-language Informed Consent Form for your study. Note that the underlined portions, in particular, will need to be tailored to your specific program and evaluation efforts. In addition, consent forms for outcome evaluation *comparison group* members should not make reference to their participation in the program being evaluated (unless they will be participating in the program at a later point in time, which should also be explained in the form).

---

### Informed Consent Form for Evaluation of [Name of Program]

**Purpose of the Study:**
I understand that in participating in [summarize the evaluation activity—e.g., a series of three surveys], I will be part of an evaluation study conducted by [name of evaluator]. The purpose of this study is to [determine the effectiveness of Program X] of [name of agency]. This study is being funded by [name of funding agency].

**Procedures:**
I understand that I will be completing a [pen and paper survey] that will ask some questions pertaining to my [knowledge, attitudes, and drug use and sexual behaviors] in relation to HIV/AIDS. I understand that [this evaluation activity] should take [approximately X minutes] to complete.

I understand that I will complete this [survey] at the following additional intervals as well: [at the end of program and at 3 and 6 months following program completion].

**Rights:**
I understand that I have the right to choose not to participate in this study. I also understand that if I do choose to participate, I have the right to refuse to answer any [survey] questions or discontinue my participation in this study at any time, without penalty. My answers to questions will not be given to anyone else, and reports or articles on the study will never identify me in any way. My participation or lack of participation in this study will not have any impact on my ability to participate in [name of program] or in other programs of the [name of agency] which I would otherwise be eligible to attend.

**Payment:**
I understand that I will receive [indicate amount of money or nature of other incentive] for the completion of [each questionnaire].

**Risks and Protections:**
I understand that the only potential risk to me in [completing this evaluation activity] is that my [survey] responses and personal information could be linked and/or made public. I understand that the evaluation staff will make every effort to prevent this from happening. This will include [describe human subjects protection security procedures used].

**Benefits of Participation:**
I understand that my participation in this study has the potential to benefit me and other clients of [name of program or agency] by providing data that can improve the quality, effectiveness, and reach of the HIV prevention-related services that are offered. I may also benefit personally by having the opportunity to assess my own [knowledge, attitudes and behaviors in regards to HIV/AIDS]. Finally, my participation may also benefit society as a whole by adding to the body of knowledge regarding the effectiveness of HIV prevention programming.

**Contact Information:**
If I would like further information on this study, I may contact [name of contact] by telephone: [phone number], email: [email address] or letter: [mailing address].

[IF APPLICABLE:] If I have concerns about this study, I may contact [name of IRB member or chair, if applicable], [member or chair] of the Institutional Review Board, by telephone: [phone number], email: [email address] or letter: [mailing address].

My signature below indicates that I agree to participate in the evaluation study, as described above.

I also understand that one copy of this Consent Form is mine to keep.

Participant's name *(please print)* _____

Participant's signature _____

Date _____

*If this document was read to the participant, the following signatures are needed:*

Witness: _____

and

Program Staff Member: _____

# Tool 4-5 Sample Informed Consent Template (Spanish)

The template below can be used to develop a Spanish-language Informed Consent Form for your study. Note that the underlined portions, in particular, will need to be tailored to your program and evaluation efforts. In addition, consent forms for outcome evaluation *comparison group* members should not make reference to their participation in the program being evaluated (unless they will be participating in the program at a later point in time, which should also be explained in the form).

---

**Forma de Permiso Informado para [Nombre del Programa]**

**Propósito del Estudio:**
Entiendo que al participar en [dé un resumen de la actividad evaluativa—p.e., tres cuestionarios) seré participante en un estudio de evaluación llevado a cabo por [nombre del evaluador] para [determinar la efectividad del Programa X] de [nombre de la agencia]. Este estudio ha sido patrocinado por [nombre de la agencia financiera].

**Procedimiento:**
Entiendo que voy a completar [una encuesta con papel y lápiz] sobre [mis conocimientos, actitudes, uso de drogas y conductas sexuales] con relación al VIH/SIDA. Entiendo que completar esta actividad requerirá [aproximadamente X minutos].

Entiendo que completaré [el cuestionario] [cuatro] veces, en total: [ahora, al fin del programa, y a los tres y los seis meses después].

**Derechos:**
Entiendo que puedo elegir a no participar en este estudio. También entiendo que si decido participar, puedo negarme a contestar cualquier pregunta [del cuestionario] o dejar de participar en el estudio en cualquier momento, sin penalización. No se compartirán mis respuestas con nadie. En ninguno de los reportes o artículos que se escriban acerca de este estudio se podrá identificarme. Mi decisión de participar or no participar en este estudio no tendrá impacto sobre mi habilidad de participar en [nombre del programa], ni en cualquier otro programa de [nombre de agencia].

**Pago:**
Entiendo que recibiré [indique cantidad de dinero u otro incentivo] por completar [cada cuestionario].

**Riesgos y Protección Contra Riesgos:**
Entiendo que el único riesgo que puedo tener al participar en este estudio es que mis respuestas y mi información personal podrían conectarse y/o hacerse públicas. Entiendo que el personal del estudio hará todo lo posible para prevenir tal ocurrencia. Esto incluirá [describa las protecciones que se emplearán].

**Beneficios de Participación:**
Entiendo que mi participación en este estudio tiene el potencial de beneficiar a mí y a los otros clientes de [nombre del programa o de la agencia], como proveeré datos que se pueden usar para mejorar la calidad, efectividad, y alcance de sus servicios para prevenir el VIH. Además, yo tal vez sacaré provecho de la oportunidad de considerar mis propios [conocimientos, actitudes, y compartimiento acerca del VIH/SIDA]. Mi participación tal vez sea beneficiosa para la sociedad en general también, porque ayudará a mejorar el conocimiento de la efectividad de programas para prevenir el VIH.

**Información de Contactos:**
Si deseo obtener más información acerca de este estudio, puedo comunicarme con [nombre] por teléfono: [número de teléfono], o por correo electrónico a: [email], o por correo a: [dirección de envío].

[SI SE APLICA:] Si tengo alguna duda o preocupación acerca de este estudio, puedo comunicarme con [nombre de miembro/a o director/a de la Junta de Revisión Institucional], [miembro/a o director/a] de la Junta de Revisión Institucional, por teléfono: [número de teléfono], o por correo electrónico a: [email], o por correo a: [dirección de envío].

Mi firma a continuación indica que estoy de acuerdo en participar en este estudio.

Una copia de esta Forma de Permiso es para mí.

Nombre del participante *(en letra de molde)* _____

Firma del participante _____

Fecha _____

*Si este documento le fue leído al participante, se requieren las siguientes firmas:*

Testigo/-a: _____

y

Personal del Programa: _____

# Tool 4-6 Oral Informed Consent Checklist

The checklist below can help you to take the steps necessary to obtain oral informed consent from evaluation participants. Place an "x" in the square box (□) as you complete each item on the list. (To do this on your computer—using the file on the CD-ROM—use your cursor to click on the box. To remove an "x" from a box, click on the box again.)

☐ 1. Develop your Informed Consent Form *(see Tools 4–4 to 4–5 for templates)* and Short Form for Oral Informed Consent *(see Tools 4–7 to 4–8 for templates)*.

☐ 2. *(If applicable:)* Obtain Institutional Review Board (IRB) approval.

☐ 3. Review your Informed Consent Form and its Short Form.
   ☐ Make sure you are familiar with the content of your forms so you can readily answer any questions that may arise.

☐ 4. Identify a witness to confirm oral presentation of informed consent.
   ☐ A witness must be present (and signature obtained) during any oral presentation and confirmation of informed consent.
   ☐ This individual can be anyone not associated with the research project (i.e., not program or evaluation staff), including another program participant.

☐ 5. Read the Short Form to the participant.

☐ 6. Read the longer Informed Consent Form to the participant.

☐ 7. Have the participant and witness sign the Short Form.
   ☐ Their signatures confirm that both forms were orally presented to the participant.
   ☐ Provide a copy of the Short Form to the participant.

☐ 8. Have the participant, witness and a program staff member sign the longer Informed Consent Form.
   ☐ Provide a copy of the Informed Consent Form to the participant.

**NOTE:** Remember that if your evaluation will involve persons under the legal age of consent (i.e., age 18 in most U.S. states), you must usually get *both* consent from the parent or guardian and assent from the minor for the minor to participate.

# Tool 4-7 Oral Informed Consent Template (Short Form, English)

The template below can be used to develop a short, English-language Oral Informed Consent Form for your study that can be used to introduce a full-length Informed Consent Form that is read to potential study participants. Note that the underlined portions, in particular, will need to be tailored to your program and evaluation efforts. In addition, consent forms for outcome evaluation *comparison group* members should not make reference to their participation in the program being evaluated (unless they will be participating in the program at a later point in time, which should also be explained in the form).

---

### Oral Informed Consent Form (Short Form) for Evaluation of [Name of Program]

You are being asked to participate in an evaluation study of [name of program] of [name of agency].

Before you can agree to participate, the evaluator must tell you about (1) the purposes, procedures, and duration of the study; (2) any reasonably foreseeable risks and benefits of the study; and (3) how your confidentiality will be maintained if you agree to participate.

The evaluator must also tell you about (1) any compensation for your participation and (2) what happens if you decide to stop participating.

If you agree to participate, you must sign and be given a copy of this document and a longer written consent form, which will be read to you. A witness will also sign both documents, to indicate that he or she has witnessed your agreement to participate.

You may contact [name] at [telephone number] any time you have questions about this study.

Your participation in this research is voluntary, and you will not be penalized or lose the opportunity to participate in the program if you refuse to participate in the study or decide to stop participating.

Signing this document means that the evaluation study, including the above information, has been described to you orally, and that you voluntarily agree to participate.

| | |
|---|---|
| _____ | _____ |
| Signature of participant | Date |
| | |
| _____ | _____ |
| Signature of witness | Date |

# Tool 4-8 Oral Informed Consent Template (Short Form, Spanish)

The template below can be used to develop a short, Spanish-language Oral Informed Consent Form for your study that can be used to introduce a full-length Informed Consent Form that is read to potential study participants. Note that the underlined portions, in particular, will need to be tailored to your program and evaluation efforts. In addition, consent forms for outcome evaluation *comparison group* members should not make reference to their participation in the program being evaluated (unless they will be participating in the program at a later point in time, which should also be explained in the form).

---

### Forma de Permiso Oral (Versión Corta) para la Evaluación de [Nombre de Programa]

Se le solicita que participe en un estudio para evaluar [nombre del programa] de [nombre de la agencia].

Antes de que Ud. pueda dar su permiso a participar, el evaluador/la evaluadora debe informarle acerca de lo siguiente: (1) el propósito, los procedimientos, y la duración del estudio; (2) cualquier riesgo o beneficio que pueda surgir como consecuencia de este estudio; y (3) cómo se va a mantener su confidencialidad.

El investigador/la investigadora también debe informarle acerca de: (1) si existe una compensación que se le dará por su participación y (2) qué ocurrirá si usted decide dejar de participar en este estudio.

Si acepta participar, debe firmar (y recibir una copia de) este documento y otro documento de permiso más largo, que se le leerá. Un/a testigo también firmará los dos documentos, para indicar que ha servido de testigo a su decisión a participar.

Si tiene preguntas acerca del estudio, puede comunicarse con [nombre] a [número de teléfono], en cualquier momento.

*Su participación en este estudio es voluntaria y no sufrirá penalización alguna, ni perderá la oportunidad de participar en el programa, si no desea participar en la evaluación o si decide dejar de participar en la evaluación una vez que haya comenzado.*

Su firma en este documento indica que se le ha explicado oralmente el estudio, incluyendo la información que aparece más arriba, y que usted acepta participar en forma voluntaria.

| | |
|---|---|
| _____ | _____ |
| Firma del participante | Fecha |
| | |
| _____ | _____ |
| Firma del/de la testigo | Fecha |

## Tool 4-9 Process Evaluation Data Collection Matrix

This matrix provides information on how to collect various types of process data. The far right column provides space for notes on your process evaluation data collection plans. To fill in the table below on your computer (using the file on your CD-ROM), click on the gray-shaded area in the box you would like to type in. (Note that the gray shading will not appear in printouts of this document.)

| Type of Data | How to Collect It | When to Collect It | Notes on Your Data Collection Plans |
|---|---|---|---|
| **1. Service Delivery** | ■ Develop **program log** forms to record services delivered *(see Tool 4–10)*.<br>■ Train staff on use of forms.<br>■ Record services delivered. | Immediately after each program session or day. | |
| **2. Participation** | ■ Collect names and basic demographic information on participants (e.g., age, race/ethnicity, gender, etc.) using a **registration form or spreadsheet**.<br>■ Assign a unique participant identifier to each participant that is tied to his/her demographic, attendance, and other information.<br>■ Create an **attendance log or spreadsheet** *(see Tool 4–11)*.<br>■ Track attendance. | At registration and after each program session or day. | |
| **3. Resource Use** | ■ Use existing **ledgers and accounting systems**, or develop new/supplemental **forms or spreadsheets** to record resource use (e.g., staff time, facilities, materials, funding).<br>■ Train staff on use of new forms or procedures (if applicable).<br>■ Record resource use. | Periodically during program implementation, as expenses are incurred. | |
| **4. Program Satisfaction**<br>■ Staff<br>■ Participant | ■ Develop **surveys** *(see Tools 4–12 to 4–13)* **or focus group or interview questions**.<br>■ Train staff on use of the instruments.<br>■ Schedule data collection points (e.g., mid-program, postprogram).<br>■ Conduct the surveys, focus groups, and/or interviews. | At the end of a program, program cycle, or client's participation in a program; for longer programs, at one or more mid-points as well. At regular intervals (e.g., every 3 or 6 months) for ongoing services that do not have cycles. | |
| **5. Cultural Competence of the Program as Implemented** | ■ Same as Row 4. | Same as Row 4. | |

# Tool 4-10 Sample Program Implementation Log

This worksheet, or an adapted version of it, can help you to assess what activities or services your program delivered, compared to what was planned.

To type directly into the various tables in the worksheet (using the file on the CD-ROM), click on the gray-shaded area in the box you would like to type in. (Note that the gray shading will not appear in printouts of this document.) To place an "x" in the checkboxes (□) using your computer, use your cursor to click on the box. To remove an "x" from a box, click on the box again.

### *Instructions*

1. In **Part I- Program Session List**, list the program name, as well as the number, name, and expected length (in minutes or hours) of each program session.
2. **Part II- Program Implementation Log** should be completed for *each* of the planned program sessions. It should be filled out by the staff member (or members) responsible for delivering the session.
   □ BEFORE each session, complete Section A of the log, "Description of Session as Planned."
   □ AFTER each session, complete Section B of the log, "Implementation of the Session," which asks *whether you implemented the session as planned or with changes*. If you *never implemented the session at all*, be sure to still complete a log for that session and check "Did not implement session." Part II also asks you to comment on your implementation experiences. It is important to fill in this information very soon after completing the session (or deciding not to implement it at all), so that your experiences are fresh in your mind.
3. The more detail that you provide in this worksheet, the more helpful the information will be in your overall evaluation of the program.

### Part I. Program Session List

| Name of Program: | |
|---|---|

**List the number (e.g., Session 1, Session 2, etc.), name, and expected length of each program session:**

| Session Number | Session Name | Expected Number of Minutes or Hours |
|---|---|---|
| | | |
| | | |
| | | |
| | | |
| | | |
| | | |
| | | |
| | | |
| | | |
| | | |
| | | |
| | | |
| | | |
| | | |
| | | |
| | | |
| | | |
| | | |
| | | |

**Part II. Program Implementation Log**

| | |
|---|---|
| **Title of Program:** | |
| **Session Number & Name:** | |
| **Expected Length:** | |
| **Name of Session Staff Member(s):** | |

**A. Description of Session as Planned.** Provide a written description of this session <u>as planned</u>, including key topics and activities that you expect to cover and delivery methods you expect to use.

 

**B. Implementation of the Session.**

*(1) Check <u>one</u> of the following:*

    ☐ Did not implement session
    ☐ Implemented session as planned
    ☐ Implemented session with changes

*(2) For this session, please describe:*

    ■ Any modifications made to the planned topics or activities.
    ■ Reasons for modifying or eliminating this session.
    ■ Reactions to this session by participants.
    ■ Any suggested changes to this session (for future implementations of the program).

# Tool 4-11 Sample Attendance Log

A worksheet like the one on the next page can help you to assess what population was reached by your program, compared to what was planned. Setting up such a worksheet in a **computerized spreadsheet program like Excel** can be particularly helpful.

**Explanation of each column in the attached sample log:**

| Column | Information in each cell of the column |
|---|---|
| ID# | A unique identification number assigned to each client or participant, to be used in lieu of their name. |
| Age | Client's age at time of enrollment. |
| Gender | Client's gender, female (F) or male (M). |
| Ethnicity | Client's ethnicity, per the ethnicity key at the bottom of the page. |
| Date | In the first row: the date of each program activity, session, meeting, or service. In the subsequent rows: a "1" in a cell means that the client whose ID number appears in the first cell of that row attended that day; a 0 in a cell means that the client did not attend that day. |
| Total attendance per person | Total number of sessions attended per person. |

**Sample Participant Attendance Log**

| ID# | Age | Gender | Ethnicity[1] | 9/15/07 | 9/22/07 | 9/29/07 | 10/6/07 | Total attendance per person |
|---|---|---|---|---|---|---|---|---|
| 123 | 16 | F | W | 1 | 1 | 1 | 0 | 3 |
| 124 | 16 | F | B | 1 | 1 | 0 | 0 | 2 |
| 125 | 15 | M | B | 1 | 1 | 1 | 1 | 4 |
| 126 | 16 | M | API | 1 | 0 | 1 | 1 | 3 |
| 127 | 15 | F | W | 0 | 1 | 1 | 0 | 2 |
| 128 | 17 | F | L | 1 | 1 | 1 | 1 | 4 |
| 129 | 17 | M | B | 1 | 1 | 0 | 1 | 3 |
| 130 | 16 | F | M | 1 | 0 | 0 | 0 | 1 |
| | | | Total attendance per session | 7 | 6 | 5 | 4 | |

[1] AI = American Indian/Native American; API = Asian/Pacific Islander; B = Black/African American; L = Latino/Hispanic; W = White/Caucasian; M = Mixed or Other

# Tool 4-12 Sample Participant Satisfaction Survey (English)

The survey below is an example of what a participant satisfaction survey focused on issues of cultural competence might look like. It can serve as a point of reference when you are designing your own participant satisfaction questionnaire(s), with your specific evaluation needs and those of your key stakeholders in mind.

---

### *Participant Satisfaction Survey*

This survey is about how [*insert name of your program*] fits your needs and how comfortable you feel with the program. This is an anonymous survey. Please be honest—your answers can help us understand what is useful about the program and what is not, and thus identify ways to improve the program to meet your needs.

Please read the statements (#1–28) below. For each statement, please check the box that best describes how you feel about the program. Then write in your answers to the last two questions (#29–30).

---

#### Satisfaction with the Program

---

1. **I feel:**
   - ☐ Very satisfied with the program
   - ☐ Somewhat satisfied with the program
   - ☐ Somewhat unsatisfied with the program
   - ☐ Very unsatisfied with the program

2a. **I would support the program.**
   - ☐ Yes      ☐ I'm not sure      ☐ No

2b. **If yes . . . I would support the program in the following ways:** *(Please check all that apply)*
   - ☐ I would publicly tell others how much I support the program
   - ☐ I would provide testimonials or support letters
   - ☐ I would provide positive feedback
   - ☐ I would come back to volunteer or work for the program
   - ☐ I would donate money to the program
   - ☐ Other_____

3a. **I have told program staff about my level of satisfaction or dissatisfaction with the program.**
   - ☐ Yes      ☐ I'm not sure      ☐ No

3b. **If yes . . . I gave my input in the following ways:** *(Please check all that apply)*
   - ☐ I was asked informally
   - ☐ I was interviewed
   - ☐ I was in a focus group
   - ☐ I put my comments in a suggestion box
   - ☐ I filled out a satisfaction survey
   - ☐ I provided a testimonial for the program
   - ☐ Other_____

---

Satisfaction with Program Staff

---

**On a scale of 1–5, with 1 being "very low" and 5 being "very high," how would you rate the following?** *(Circle one answer for each item.)*

|  | *Very Low* . . . . . . . . . . . . . . . . *Very High* |  |  |  |  |  |
|---|---|---|---|---|---|---|
| 4. Staff members' level of training to serve people like me | 1 | 2 | 3 | 4 | 5 | Not sure |
| 5. Program staff's ability to talk about diversity within my community | 1 | 2 | 3 | 4 | 5 | Not sure |
| 6. Program staff's knowledge about the cultural, social, and religious beliefs of my community | 1 | 2 | 3 | 4 | 5 | Not sure |
| 7. Program staff's ability to discuss HIV/AIDS in a culturally sensitive way | 1 | 2 | 3 | 4 | 5 | Not sure |
| 8. My level of comfort in talking with program staff | 1 | 2 | 3 | 4 | 5 | Not sure |
| 9. Program staff's ability to handle disagreement within a group | 1 | 2 | 3 | 4 | 5 | Not sure |

---

Satisfaction with Language Use

---

**On a scale of 1–5, with 1 being "very low" and 5 being "very high," how would you rate the following?** *(Circle one answer for each item.)*

|  | *Very Low* . . . . . . . . . . . . . . . . *Very High* |  |  |  |  |  |
|---|---|---|---|---|---|---|
| 10. My understanding of the language in the program materials | 1 | 2 | 3 | 4 | 5 | Not sure |
| 11. My level of comfort with the language in the program materials | 1 | 2 | 3 | 4 | 5 | Not sure |
| 12. Program staff members' language abilities and skills in interacting with me | 1 | 2 | 3 | 4 | 5 | Not sure |

13a. **I have given input to program staff about my language needs and how I am most comfortable communicating.**
  □ Yes  □ I'm not sure  □ No

13b. **If yes . . . I gave my input in the following ways:** *(Please check all that apply)*
  □ I was asked informally  □ I filled out a satisfaction survey
  □ I was interviewed  □ I helped the program test existing materials
  □ I was in a focus group  □ Other＿＿＿＿＿＿
  □ I put my comments in a suggestion box

14. **I was asked by the program whether staff members have the language abilities and skills to serve me well.**
  □ Yes  □ I'm not sure  □ No

14b. **If yes . . . I gave my input in the following ways:** *(Please check all that apply)*
  □ I was asked informally  □ I put my comments/opinions in a suggestion box
  □ I was interviewed  □ I filled out a satisfaction survey
  □ I was in a focus group  □ Other＿＿＿＿＿＿

Satisfaction with Program Fit

**On a scale of 1–5, with 1 being "very low" and 5 being "very high," how would you rate the following?** *(Circle one answer for each item.)*

| | Very Low | | | | Very High | |
|---|---|---|---|---|---|---|
| 15. Program staff's understanding of the importance of making the program work for the people who use it | 1 | 2 | 3 | 4 | 5 | Not sure |
| 16. My understanding of the information the program presents | 1 | 2 | 3 | 4 | 5 | Not sure |
| 17. The fit of the program materials with my ideas and beliefs. | 1 | 2 | 3 | 4 | 5 | Not sure |
| 18. My level of comfort with the examples, pictures, and stories used by the program | 1 | 2 | 3 | 4 | 5 | Not sure |
| 19. The degree to which the program uses situations that seem realistic to me | 1 | 2 | 3 | 4 | 5 | Not sure |
| 20. The degree to which the program talks about issues and problems that my community faces | 1 | 2 | 3 | 4 | 5 | Not sure |
| 21. The degree to which the program talks about why it can be hard to think about HIV prevention | 1 | 2 | 3 | 4 | 5 | Not sure |
| 22. The degree to which the program talks about differences that exist between people within my community | 1 | 2 | 3 | 4 | 5 | Not sure |

23a. **I have given input to program staff about cultural, religious, social, and economic issues that are important to me.**
  ☐ Yes          ☐ I'm not sure          ☐ No

23b. **If yes ... I gave my input in the following ways:** *(Please check all that apply)*
  ☐ I was asked informally                    ☐ I put my comments/opinions in a suggestion box
  ☐ I was interviewed                          ☐ I filled out a satisfaction survey
  ☐ I was in a focus group                     ☐ Other_____

24a. **I have given input to program staff about who my community leaders are.**
  ☐ Yes          ☐ I'm not sure          ☐ No

24b. **If yes ... I gave my input in the following ways:** *(Please check all that apply)*
  ☐ I was asked informally                    ☐ I put my comments/opinions in a suggestion box
  ☐ I was interviewed                          ☐ I filled out a satisfaction survey
  ☐ I was in a focus group                     ☐ Other_____

25a. **I have given input to program staff on how to make it easier for people to get to and use the program.**
  ☐ Yes          ☐ I'm not sure          ☐ No

25b. **If yes ... I gave my input in the following ways:** *(Please check all that apply)*
  ☐ I was asked informally                    ☐ I put my comments/opinions in a suggestion box
  ☐ I was interviewed                          ☐ I filled out a satisfaction survey
  ☐ I was in a focus group                     ☐ Other_____

26a. **I have given input to program staff about how well the program fits with my cultural, religious, and social beliefs.**
  ☐ Yes          ☐ I'm not sure          ☐ No

26b. **If yes … I gave my input in the following ways:** *(Please check all that apply)*
    ☐ I was asked informally          ☐ I put my comments/opinions in a suggestion box
    ☐ I was interviewed               ☐ I filled out a satisfaction survey
    ☐ I was in a focus group           ☐ Other_____

27. **The program made changes to improve the fit with my cultural, religious and social beliefs.**
    ☐ Yes          ☐ I'm not sure          ☐ No

28. **The program made changes in order to make it easier for people to get to and use the program.**
    ☐ Yes          ☐ I'm not sure          ☐ No

29. **Other ways in which the program paid attention to issues that are important to me include:**

_____

_____

_____

30. **Other ways in which the program should pay more attention to issues that are important to me include:**

_____

_____

_____

THANK YOU FOR YOUR PARTICIPATION!

# Tool 4-13 Sample Participant Satisfaction Survey (Spanish)

The survey below is an example of what a participant satisfaction survey focused on issues of cultural competence might look like. It can serve as a point of reference when you are designing your own participant satisfaction questionnaire(s), with your specific evaluation needs and those of your key stakeholders in mind.

---

### *Cuestionario sobre Satisfacción con el Programa*

Este cuestionario tiene como propósito ver cómo [*nombre de su programa*] corresponde a sus necesidades y cómo se siente en relación al programa. Le pedimos que conteste en forma honesta – sus respuestas nos ayudarán a entender mejor lo que sirve y lo que no sirve del programa, y cómo podemos mejorar el programa para mejor servir a nuestros clientes.

Lea las oraciones (#1-28) que aparecen a continuación. Para cada una de ellas, marque la cajita que mejor describe lo que Ud. piensa del programa. Para #29-30, indique sus respuestas en sus propias palarabras.

---

Satisfacción con el Programa

---

**1. Estoy:**
- ☐ Muy satisfecho/a con el programa
- ☐ Algo satisfecho/a con el programa
- ☐ Algo insatisfecho/a con el programa
- ☐ Muy insatisfecho/a con el programa

**2a. Le daría mi apoyo al programa.**
- ☐ Sí          ☐ No estoy seguro/a          ☐ No

**2b. Si mi respuesta es afirmativa... apoyaría al programa de la(s) forma(s) siguiente(s):** *(Marque todas las respuestas que correspondan)*
- ☐ Le diría a otros en forma pública cuánto apoyo el programa
- ☐ Proveería testimonios o cartas de apoyo
- ☐ Haría comentarios positivos
- ☐ Volvería como voluntario/a o trabajaría para el programa
- ☐ Daría dinero para el programa
- ☐ Otra forma_____

**3a. He informado al personal del programa sobre mi satisfacción o descontento con el programa.**
- ☐ Sí          ☐ No estoy seguro/a          ☐ No

**3b. Si mi respuesta es afirmativa... hice mis comentarios de las siguientes formas:** *(Marque todas las respuestas que correspondan)*
- ☐ Me preguntaron de forma informal
- ☐ Me entrevistaron
- ☐ Participé en un grupo de enfoque ("focus group")
- ☐ Puse mis comentarios en una caja de sugerencias
- ☐ Llené una encuesta de satisfacción
- ☐ Di un testimonio sobre el programa
- ☐ Otra forma_____

---

Satisfacción con el personal del programa

---

**En una escala de 1 a 5, en que "1" quiere decir "muy bajo/a" y "5" quiere decir "muy alto/a," ¿cómo calificaría cada una de las oraciones siguientes?** *(Marque una respuesta para cada oración.)*

| | *Muy*<br>*Bajo/a* .............. | | | *Muy*<br>*Alto/a* | | |
|---|---|---|---|---|---|---|
| 4. El nivel de entrenamiento/capacitación del personal del programa para servir a gente como yo | 1 | 2 | 3 | 4 | 5 | No estoy seguro/a |
| 5. La capacidad del personal del programa para hablar de diversidad en mi comunidad | 1 | 2 | 3 | 4 | 5 | No estoy seguro/a |
| 6. El conocimento del personal del programa acerca de las creencias culturales, sociales y religiosas de mi comunidad | 1 | 2 | 3 | 4 | 5 | No estoy seguro/a |
| 7. La capacidad del personal del programa de hablar del VIH/SIDA en una forma apropiada para mi cultura | 1 | 2 | 3 | 4 | 5 | No estoy seguro/a |
| 8. Mi nivel de comodidad al hablar con personal del programa | 1 | 2 | 3 | 4 | 5 | No estoy seguro/a |
| 9. La capacidad del personal del programa de enfrentar desacuerdos dentro de un grupo | 1 | 2 | 3 | 4 | 5 | No estoy seguro/a |

---

Satisfacción con el uso de lenguaje

---

**En una escala de 1 a 5, en que "1" quiere decir "muy bajo/a" y "5" quiere decir "muy alto/a," ¿cómo calificaría cada una de las oraciones siguientes?** *(Marque una respuesta para cada oración.)*

| | *Muy*<br>*Bajo/a* .............. | | | *Muy*<br>*Alto/a* | | |
|---|---|---|---|---|---|---|
| 10. Mi entendimiento del lenguaje en el material del programa | 1 | 2 | 3 | 4 | 5 | No estoy seguro/a |
| 11. Mi nivel de comodidad con el lenguaje en el material del programa | 1 | 2 | 3 | 4 | 5 | No estoy seguro/a |
| 12. Las habilidades lingüísticas del personal del programa cuando hablan conmigo | 1 | 2 | 3 | 4 | 5 | No estoy seguro/a |

**13a.** He informado al personal del programa sobre mis necesidades en cuanto al lenguaje y cómo prefiero comunicar.
☐ Sí          ☐ No estoy seguro/a          ☐ No

**13b.** Si mi respuesta es afirmativa . . . hice mis comentarios de la(s) siguiente(s) forma(s): *(Marque todas las respuestas que correspondan)*
☐ Me preguntaron de forma informal          ☐ Puse mis comentarios en una caja de sugerencias
☐ Me entrevistaron          ☐ Llené una encuesta de satisfacción
☐ Participé en un grupo de enfoque          ☐ Ayudé al programa probar sus materiales
("focus group")          ☐ Otra forma_____

**14a.** Me preguntó alguien del personal del programa si el personal tiene las habilidades lingüísticas y las aptitudes necesarias para servirme bien.
☐ Sí          ☐ No estoy seguro/a          ☐ No

**14b. Si mi respuesta es afirmativa... hice mis comentarios de la(s) siguiente(s) forma(s):** *(Marque todas las respuestas que correspondan)*

☐ Me preguntaron de forma informal
☐ Me entrevistaron
☐ Participé en un grupo de enfoque ("focus group)

☐ Puse mis comentarios en una caja de sugerencias
☐ Llené una encuesta de satisfacción
☐ Otra forma_____

---

Satisfacción acerca de cómo el programa se adecua a mis necesidades

---

**En una escala de 1 a 5, en que "1" quiere decir "muy bajo/a" y "5" quiere decir "muy alto/a," ¿cómo calificaría cada una de las oraciones siguientes?** *(Marque una respuesta para cada oración.)*

| | *Muy Bajo/a............... Muy Alto/a* | | | | | |
|---|---|---|---|---|---|---|
| 15. El entendimiento del personal del programa de la importancia de que el programa funcione para las personas que lo usan | 1 | 2 | 3 | 4 | 5 | No estoy seguro/a |
| 16. Mi entendimiento de la información que el programa presenta | 1 | 2 | 3 | 4 | 5 | No estoy seguro/a |
| 17. El grado de correspondencia de los materiales del programa con mis ideas y creencias | 1 | 2 | 3 | 4 | 5 | No estoy seguro/a |
| 18. Mi nivel de comodidad con los ejemplos, imágenes, e historias que el programa usa | 1 | 2 | 3 | 4 | 5 | No estoy seguro/a |
| 19. La frecuencia con que el programa usa situaciones que me parecen realistas | 1 | 2 | 3 | 4 | 5 | No estoy seguro/a |
| 20. La frecuencia con que el programa trata temas y problemas que enfrentan mi comunidad | 1 | 2 | 3 | 4 | 5 | No estoy seguro/a |
| 21. La frecuencia con que el programa trata por qué puede ser difícil pensar en la prevención del VIH | 1 | 2 | 3 | 4 | 5 | No estoy seguro/a |
| 22. La frecuencia con que el programa trata las diferencias que existen entre personas de mi comunidad | 1 | 2 | 3 | 4 | 5 | No estoy seguro/a |

**23a. He informado al personal del programa sobre los aspectos culturales, religiosos, sociales y económicos que son importantes para mí.**

☐ Sí          ☐ No estoy seguro/a          ☐ No

**23b. Si mi respuesta es afirmativa... hice mis comentarios de la(s) siguiente(s) forma(s):** *(Marque todas las respuestas que correspondan)*

☐ Me preguntaron de forma informal
☐ Me entrevistaron
☐ Participé en un grupo de enfoque ("focus group")

☐ Puse mis comentarios en una caja de sugerencias
☐ Llené una encuesta de satisfacción
☐ Otra forma_____

**24a. He informado al personal del programa sobre quiénes son los líderes de mi comunidad.**

☐ Sí          ☐ No estoy seguro/a          ☐ No

**24b. Si mi respuesta es afirmativa... hice mis comentarios de la(s) siguiente(s) forma(s):** *(Marque todas las respuestas que correspondan)*

☐ Me preguntaron de forma informal
☐ Me entrevistaron
☐ Participé en un grupo de enfoque ("focus group")

☐ Puse mis comentarios en una caja de sugerencias
☐ Llené una encuesta de satisfacción
☐ Otra forma_____

**25a. He hablado con el personal del programa sobre la manera de facilitar el acceso al programa y el uso del programa para la gente.**

☐ Sí            ☐ No estoy seguro/a            ☐ No

**25b. Si mi respuesta es afirmativa...hice mis comentarios de la(s) siguiente(s) forma(s):** *(Marque todas las respuestas que correspondan)*

☐ Me preguntaron de forma informal            ☐ Puse mis comentarios en una caja de sugerencias

☐ Me entrevistaron            ☐ Llené una encuesta de satisfacción

☐ Participé en un grupo de enfoque ("focus group")            ☐ Otra forma_____

**26a. He hablado con el personal del programa sobre el grado de correspondencia del programa con mis creencias culturales, religiosas y sociales.**

☐ Sí            ☐ No estoy seguro/a            ☐ No

**26b. Si mi respuesta es afirmativa...hice mis comentarios de la(s) siguiente(s) forma(s)** *(Marque todas las respuestas que correspondan)*

☐ Me preguntaron de forma informal            ☐ Puse mis comentarios en una caja de sugerencias

☐ Me entrevistaron            ☐ Llené una encuesta de satisfacción

☐ Participé en un grupo de enfoque ("focus group")            ☐ Otra forma_____

**27. El programa hizo cambios para corresponder mejor a mis creencias culturales, religiosas y sociales.**

☐ Sí            ☐ No estoy seguro/a            ☐ No

**28. El programa hizo cambios para facilitar el acceso y el uso para la gente.**

☐ Sí            ☐ No estoy seguro/a            ☐ No

**29. Otras maneras en que el programa prestó atención a lo que es importante para mí:**

_____

_____

**30. Otras maneras en que el programa debería prestar más atención a lo que es importante para mí:**

_____

_____

¡MUCHAS GRACIAS POR SU PARTICIPACIÓN!

# Tool 4-14 Outcome Evaluation Readiness Screening Checklist[1]

The worksheet below will help you to assess the readiness of your program for a culturally competent outcome evaluation. To place an "x" in the checkboxes (□) on your computer (using the file on the CD-ROM), use your cursor to click on the box. To remove an "x" from a box, click on the box again. To type into the "Notes" column, click on the gray-shaded area in the box you wish to type in. (Note that the gray shading will not appear in printouts of this document.)

## 1. Strength of program design

| Criteria | Notes |
|---|---|
| □ a. To what extent does the program address HIV-related needs and assets of the target population, local community, and agency? | |
| □ b. How robustly are cultural factors influencing HIV risk addressed? | |
| □ c. Is the program consistent with local cultural norms? | |
| □ d. Does the program design present a coherent theory of change? | |
| □ e. How strong are links among program components, objectives, and goals? | |
| □ f. How robustly does the program incorporate characteristics common to effective programs? | |
| □ g. Is there consensus on the design among key stakeholders? | |
| □ h. Is there a written program model (logic model) that provides a visual representation of the program's theory of change? | |

## 2. Strength of program implementation

| Criteria | Notes |
|---|---|
| □ a. Do your process evaluation results indicate that your program has been implemented as planned? | |
| □ b. Do your process evaluation results indicate that your program has been reaching the intended target audience? | |
| □ c. Do you process evaluation results indicate strong client satisfaction with the program? | |
| □ d. Do you process evaluation results indicate strong staff satisfaction with the program? | |
| □ e. Do you process evaluation results indicate that the program is being implemented in a culturally competent manner? | |

---

[1] Based in part on: (a) Kirby, D. (2004). BDI logic models: A useful tool for designing, strengthening, and evaluating programs to reduce adolescent sexual risk-taking, pregnancy, HIV, and other STDs. Retrieved July 3, 2005, from http://www.etr.org/recapp/BDILOGICMODEL20030924.pdf (b) Sedivy, V. (2000). *Evaluation readiness assessment guide: Is your program ready to evaluate its effectiveness?* Los Altos, CA: Sociometrics Corporation.

## 3. Accessibility of program and comparison group participants

| Criteria | Notes |
|---|---|
| ☐ a. How mobile is your population? | |
| ☐ b. What is your program drop-out rate? | |
| ☐ c. How "captive" are your participants (e.g., are they in school, prison, military, homeless)? | |
| ☐ d. How easy or difficult would it be to track your participants (e.g., through contact with their relatives, friends, etc.)? | |
| ☐ e. What kinds of incentives would be needed to retain participants in your evaluation study? | |

## 4. Resource availability

| Criteria | Notes |
|---|---|
| ☐ a. What amount of funding is available for outcome evaluation? | |
| ☐ b. What staff expertise (including employees, consultants, student interns, and volunteers) is available for:<br>■ Evaluation design<br>■ Instrument development<br>■ Data collection<br>■ Data entry<br>■ Data analysis<br>■ Report writing | |
| ☐ Do staff have the time and commitment needed to engage in outcome evaluation activities? | |
| ☐ What resources are available for participant incentives? | |
| ☐ What computer resources, office equipment, and existing data collection instruments are available for outcome evaluation? | |
| ☐ Are the available funding and other resources sufficient to support the activities needed to answer your outcome evaluation questions? | |
| ☐ Is there time during the course of your program to involve participants in evaluation activities without compromising program participation or engagement? | |

## 5. Ability to engage stakeholders

| Criteria | Notes |
|---|---|
| ☐ Are community leaders or other members interested in and available to participate in outcome evaluation design, implementation, and results dissemination? | |
| ☐ Are program staff and management in favor of involving other community leaders/members actively in evaluation design, implementation, and results dissemination? | |
| ☐ Is a plan in place to involve community leaders/members actively in evaluation design, implementation, and results dissemination? | |
| ☐ Can the multiple visions for outcome evaluation—i.e., those of program staff, management, funders, community members, and other stakeholders—be reconciled? | |

# Tool 4-15 Sample Evaluation Outcome Survey (English)

The sample outcome evaluation survey below can serve as a point of reference when you are designing your own outcome evaluation survey. Your survey should reflect the goals and objectives of your program and the cultural and linguistic background(s) of participants.

*Sample Outcome Survey*

**Thank you for participating in this evaluation study. Please answer the following questions as honestly as you can. Your responses will help us to understand how effective the program is and make it even more effective for people such as yourself.**

1. **What is your sex?** *(Please select only one answer)*
   ☐ Male
   ☐ Female
   ☐ Transsexual *(someone who is in the process, or completed the process, of changing his/her sex . . . if you check this box, please specify by checking a box below)*
      ☐ Male-to-female
      ☐ Female-to-male

2. **What is your current age?**
   _____years old

3. **What is the highest educational level you ever completed?** *(Please select only one answer)*
   ☐ Less than high school
   ☐ High school graduate
   ☐ Some college
   ☐ College graduate
   ☐ Postgraduate

4. **Which of the following best describes your current employment status?** *(Please select only one answer)*
   ☐ Employed full-time
   ☐ Employed part-time
   ☐ Stay-at-home parent
   ☐ Not currently working
   ☐ Retired

5. **Which of the following categories best represents the total income for everyone living in your home?** *(Please select only one answer)*
   ☐ Less than $10,000 per year
   ☐ $10,000–$15,000 per year
   ☐ $15,000–$25,000 per year
   ☐ $25,000–$50,000 per year
   ☐ $50,000–$75,000 per year
   ☐ Over $75,000 per year

6. **What is your current relationship status?** *(Please select only one answer)*
   ☐ Living together with a spouse/partner
   ☐ Have a spouse/partner but not living with him/her
   ☐ Neither married nor in a relationship with a partner

7. **Do you have any living children (including adopted or step-children)?** *(Please select only one answer)*
   ☐ Yes, I have_____number of living children
   ☐ No

8. **Have you ever been tested for HIV/AIDS?** *(Note: donating blood is not the same thing as getting tested for HIV/AIDS) (Please select only one answer)*
   ☐ Yes, the date of last testing was: Month_____ Year_____
   ☐ If yes, did you receive your results? ☐ Yes ☐ No
   ☐ No, I have never been tested for HIV/AIDS

9. **Please indicate whether you agree or disagree with each statement by circling the number that corresponds to your answer:**

| | Agree | Disagree | Don't Know |
|---|---|---|---|
| a. There is a difference between having the HIV virus and having the AIDS disease. | 1 | 2 | 3 |
| b. AIDS is a disease which affects only homosexual or gay men. | 1 | 2 | 3 |
| c. There is no known cure for AIDS at the present time. | 1 | 2 | 3 |
| d. Contraceptives other than condoms (such as birth control pills, diaphragms, spermicidal jelly/foam/cream) are effective in preventing the transmission of HIV. | 1 | 2 | 3 |
| e. There is no risk of transmitting HIV in sharing needles with someone else for drug use. | 1 | 2 | 3 |
| f. HIV cripples the body's natural protection against diseases. | 1 | 2 | 3 |
| g. HIV can be passed on during sexual intercourse (vaginal, anal, oral). | 1 | 2 | 3 |
| h. A pregnant woman with the HIV virus can pass it on to her baby. | 1 | 2 | 3 |
| i. Condoms are not effective in preventing the transmission of HIV during sex. | 1 | 2 | 3 |

10. **Please indicate how likely you think it is that a person can get AIDS by engaging in the following activities:**

| | Very Likely (almost certain) | Good Chance | 50–50 Chance | Some Chance | Very Unlikely (almost impossible) | Don't Know |
|---|---|---|---|---|---|---|
| a. Shaking hands or touching someone who has AIDS | 1 | 2 | 3 | 4 | 5 | 6 |
| b. Kissing someone who has AIDS | 1 | 2 | 3 | 4 | 5 | 6 |
| c. Sharing plates/forks/ glasses with someone who has AIDS | 1 | 2 | 3 | 4 | 5 | 6 |
| d. Using public bathrooms | 1 | 2 | 3 | 4 | 5 | 6 |
| e. Being coughed or sneezed on by someone who has AIDS | 1 | 2 | 3 | 4 | 5 | 6 |
| f. Working near someone who has AIDS | 1 | 2 | 3 | 4 | 5 | 6 |

---

**The following questions are about your use of drugs for pleasure, rather than medical use.**

---

11. **Have you ever taken any drugs using a needle? This includes injecting intravenously, muscling, or skin-popping. *(Please select only one answer)***
    ☐ Yes
    ☐ No *(If No, please skip to Question #16)*

12. **In the past 3 months, have you even once shot drugs with a needle that someone else had used without first cleaning it with bleach? *(Please select only one answer)***
    ☐ Yes, I have done this_____number of times
    ☐ No *(If No, please skip to Question #14)*

13. **In the past 3 months, with how many different people, if any, have you shared needles without first cleaning the needles with bleach?**
    _____Number of people

14. **In the past 3 months, did you share a cotton, cooker, or rinse water with another injection drug user?** *(Please select only one answer)*
    ☐ Yes, I have done this_____number of times
    ☐ No

15. **In the past 3 months, have you shared injection drugs by "frontloading" or "backloading?"** *(Please select only one answer)*
    ☐ Yes, I have done this_____number of times
    ☐ No

16. **In general, are you sexually attracted to:** *(Please select only one answer)*
    ☐ Only men
    ☐ Mostly men
    ☐ Both men and women
    ☐ Mostly women
    ☐ Only women
    ☐ I don't know

17. **Do you think of yourself as:** *(Please select only one answer)*
    ☐ Heterosexual
    ☐ Homosexual
    ☐ Bisexual
    ☐ Something else *(please specify)*_____
    ☐ I don't know

---

For the rest of the questions in this survey, we ask about oral, anal, and vaginal sex. Please see below for definitions of each.

*Oral sex = mouth on vagina, penis, or anus*

*Anal sex = penis in anus*

*Vaginal sex = penis in vagina*

---

18. **Have you had sexual intercourse (vaginal, oral, or anal) with either men or women in the past 3 months?** *(Please select only one answer)*
    ☐ Yes
    ☐ No  *(if No, please skip to question #26)*

19. **How many different sexual partners have you had in the past 3 months?** *(Please select only one answer)*
    ☐ 1
    ☐ 2
    ☐ 3
    ☐ 4
    ☐ 5–10
    ☐ 11–20
    ☐ 21–50
    ☐ 51 or more

20. **In the past 3 months, have you exchanged sex for money, drugs or other goods or services?**
    ☐ Yes
    ☐ No

21. **How many times in the past 3 months have you had sex while you or your partner was feeling the effects of alcohol or drugs (such as marijuana, cocaine, heroin, or crack)?**
    _____Number of times

22. **How many MALE sexual partners, if any, have you had sex with in the past 3 months?**
    _____Number of male partners *(if number of male partners is 0, skip to Question #24)*

23. **Please circle the number that indicates how many times in the past 3 months you have engaged in each of the following activities with your MALE sexual partner(s):**
    *(if you are male, please skip Item #a about penile-vaginal intercourse)*

|  | Have not engaged in this sex act in the past 3 months | 0 Times | 1–5 Times | 6–10 Times | 11–20 Times | 21–50 Times | 51+ Times |
|---|---|---|---|---|---|---|---|
| a. Penile-vaginal intercourse without a condom | 1 | 2 | 3 | 4 | 5 | 6 | 7 |
| b. Penile-anal intercourse without a condom | 1 | 2 | 3 | 4 | 5 | 6 | 7 |
| c. Oral sex (where you performed on partner) without a condom, dental dam or non-microwavable plastic wrap | 1 | 2 | 3 | 4 | 5 | 6 | 7 |

24. **How many FEMALE sexual partners, if any, have you had sex with in the past 3 months?**
    _____ Number of female partners *(if number of female partners is 0, skip to question #26*

25. **Please circle the number that indicates how many times in the past 3 months you have engaged in each of the following activities with your FEMALE sexual partner(s):**
    *(If you are female, please skip Item #a about penile-vaginal intercourse and Item #b about penile-anal intercourse)*

|  | Have not engaged in this sex act in the past 3 months | 0 Times | 1–5 Times | 6–10 Times | 11–20 Times | 21–50 Times | 51+ Times |
|---|---|---|---|---|---|---|---|
| a. Penile-vaginal intercourse without a condom | 1 | 2 | 3 | 4 | 5 | 6 | 7 |
| b. Penile-anal intercourse without a condom | 1 | 2 | 3 | 4 | 5 | 6 | 7 |
| c. Oral sex (where you performed on partner) without a condom, dental dam or non-microwavable plastic wrap | 1 | 2 | 3 | 4 | 5 | 6 | 7 |

**26.** **Are you Hispanic or Latino?** (*Please select only one answer*)

☐ Yes
☐ No

**27.** **Most people think of themselves as belonging to a particular racial group. Which of the following do you belong to?**

☐ White
☐ Native Alaskan
☐ Native Hawaiian
☐ Native American/American Indian
☐ African American
☐ Other Black
☐ Asian/Asian American
☐ Pacific Islander
☐ Mixed Race *(please specify)* _____
☐ Other *(please specify)* _____

**28.** **For each of the following activities, please indicate which language you are most comfortable using:**

|  | Only English | Mostly English | Both English and Other Language(s) Equally | Mostly Another/Other Language(s) | Only Another/Other Language(s) |
|---|---|---|---|---|---|
| a. When talking with close friends | 1 | 2 | 3 | 4 | 5 |
| b. When talking with family at home | 1 | 2 | 3 | 4 | 5 |
| c. When reading books, magazines, papers | 1 | 2 | 3 | 4 | 5 |
| d. When listening to the radio | 1 | 2 | 3 | 4 | 5 |

**29.** **If you use a language other than English at all, what is/are the language(s)?** _____

**YOU ARE NOW AT THE END OF THE SURVEY.**
***THANK YOU* FOR HAVING FILLED IT OUT.**

# Tool 4-16 Sample Evaluation Outcome Survey (Spanish)

The survey below is an example of what an outcome evaluation survey might look like. It can serve as a point of reference when your are designing your own outcome evaluation survey, with the needs of key stakeholders and the backgrounds of your clients in mind

### *Ejemplo de un Cuestionario Sobre Resultados*

**Muchas gracias por su participación en este estudio evaluativo. Por favor conteste las preguntas siguientes tan honestamente como pueda. Sus respuestas nos ayudarán a entender qué tan efectivo sea nuestro programa y cómo podemos mejorar su efectividad.**

1. **¿Cuál es su sexo?** *(Por favor seleccione una sola respuesta)*
   - ☐ Masculino
   - ☐ Femenino
   - ☐ Transexual *(alguien que está en proceso, o que ha completado el proceso de cambiar de sexo... Si usted selecciona esta respuesta, por favor especifique su respuesta al marcar una de las siguientes dos opciones)*
     - ☐ masculino-a-femenino
     - ☐ femenino-a-masculino

2. **¿Cuál es su edad?**
   - _____ **años de edad**

3. **¿Cuál es el nivel de educación más alto que ha completado?** *(Por favor seleccione una sola respuesta)*
   - ☐ No completé la escuela secundaria
   - ☐ Me gradué de la escuela secundaria
   - ☐ Algunos cursos en la universidad
   - ☐ Me gradué de la universidad
   - ☐ Hice estudios de post-grado

4. **¿Cuál de las respuestas siguientes describe mejor su situación de empleo actual?** *(Por favor seleccione una sola respuesta)*
   - ☐ Empleado/a a tiempo completo
   - ☐ Empleado/a a medio tiempo
   - ☐ Padre/madre que se dedica exclusivamente al cuidado de los niños
   - ☐ No estoy trabajando actualmente
   - ☐ Jubilado/a

5. **¿Cuál de las categorías siguientes representa mejor el ingreso total de las personas que viven en su hogar?** *(Por favor seleccione una sola respuesta)*
   - ☐ Menos de $10,000 por año
   - ☐ $10,000–$15,000 por año
   - ☐ $15,000–$25,000 por año
   - ☐ $25,000–$50,000 por año
   - ☐ $50,000–$75,000 por año
   - ☐ Más de $75,000 por año

6. **¿Cuál es su estado actual?** *(Por favor seleccione una sola respuesta)*
   - ☐ Casado/a o viviendo con su pareja
   - ☐ Tiene esposo/a o pareja pero no vive con él/ella
   - ☐ No tiene ni esposo/a ni pareja

7. **¿Tiene hijos vivos (incluyendo a los hijos/as adoptados/as o políticos/as)?** *(Por favor seleccione una sola respuesta)*
   - ☐ Sí, tengo_____hijos/as vivos/as
   - ☐ No

8. **¿Se le ha hecho alguna vez la prueba de VIH?** *(Donar sangre no es lo mismo que hacer la prueba de VIH.)* *(Por favor seleccione una sola respuesta)*
   - ☐ Sí, la fecha de la última prueba fue: Mes_____Año_____
   - ☐ Si responde en forma afirmativa, ¿recibió los resultados? ☐ Sí ☐ No
   - ☐ No, nunca me hicieron la prueba de VIH

9. **Por favor indique si está o no está de acuerdo con cada una de las oraciones que aparecen a continuación. Marque su respuesta con un círculo:**

| | Estoy de acuerdo | No estoy de acuerdo | No sé |
|---|---|---|---|
| a. Hay una diferencia entre tener el virus de VIH y tener la enfermedad de SIDA. | 1 | 2 | 3 |
| b. El SIDA es una enfermedad que afecta únicamente a los hombres homosexuales o a los "gays." | 1 | 2 | 3 |
| c. Hasta ahora no se ha descubierto una cura para el SIDA. | 1 | 2 | 3 |
| d. Los anticonceptivos que no sean condones (como por ejemplo la píldora, el diafragma, los espermicidas en forma de espuma, crema, o gel) son efectivos para impedir la transmisión del VIH. | 1 | 2 | 3 |
| e. No existe ningún riesgo de transmisión de VIH si se comparten agujas con alguien para inyectar drogas. | 1 | 2 | 3 |
| f. El VIH anula la protección natural que el cuerpo humano tiene contra las enfermedades. | 1 | 2 | 3 |
| g. El VIH puede transmitirse durante las relaciones sexuales (ya sea por vía vaginal, anal, u oral). | 1 | 2 | 3 |
| h. Una mujer embarazada que tenga el virus de VIH puede transmitírselo al bebé. | 1 | 2 | 3 |
| i. Los condones no son efectivos para prevenir la transmisión del VIH durante las relaciones sexuales. | 1 | 2 | 3 |

10. **Por favor indique qué posibilidades tiene una persona de contraer SIDA al hacer las actividades siguientes:**

| | Es muy probable (casi seguro) | Tiene buena proba-bilidad | 50-50 de proba-bilidad | Alguna proba-bilidad | No es muy probable (casi imposible) | No sé |
|---|---|---|---|---|---|---|
| a. Dar la mano, o tocar, a alguien que tiene SIDA | 1 | 2 | 3 | 4 | 5 | 6 |
| b. Besar a alguien que tiene SIDA | 1 | 2 | 3 | 4 | 5 | 6 |
| c. Compartir platos/tenedores/vasos con alguien que tiene SIDA | 1 | 2 | 3 | 4 | 5 | 6 |
| d. Usar baños públicos | 1 | 2 | 3 | 4 | 5 | 6 |
| e. Si alguien que tiene SIDA le tose o estornuda encima | 1 | 2 | 3 | 4 | 5 | 6 |
| f. Trabajar cerca de alguien que tiene SIDA | 1 | 2 | 3 | 4 | 5 | 6 |

---

**Las preguntas siguientes se refieren al uso de drogas para fines de placer, no para fines médicos.**

---

11. **¿Se ha drogado alguna vez usando una aguja? Esto incluye el inyectarse en forma intravenosa, sobre músculo o intra-dérmica.** *(Por favor seleccione una sola respuesta)*
    - ☐ Sí
    - ☐ No *(Si responde "No", por favor pase a la pregunta No. 16)*

12. **En los últimos 3 meses, ¿se ha drogado al menos una vez con la aguja que otra persona había usado sin primero limpiarlo con cloro?** *(Por favor seleccione una sola respuesta)*
    - ☐ Sí, he hecho esto_____veces *(indique número de veces)*
    - ☐ No *(Si responde "No", por favor pase a la pregunta No. 14)*

13. En los últimos 3 meses, ¿con cuántas personas diferentes ha compartido agujas sin primero limpiarlas con cloro?

    _____*(indique el número de personas)*

14. En los últimos 3 meses, ¿ha compartido un trozo de algodón, un hervidor, o el agua de enjuague con otra persona que también se inyecta drogas? *(Por favor seleccione una sola respuesta)*

    ☐ Sí, lo he hecho_____veces *(indique el número de veces)*
    ☐ No

15. En los últimos 3 meses, ¿ha compartido drogas inyectadas haciendo "frontloading" or "backloading" (usando dos jeringas)? *(Por favor seleccione una sola respuesta)*

    ☐ Sí, lo he hecho_____veces *(indique el número de veces)*
    ☐ No

16. Por lo general, a usted le atraen: *(Por favor seleccione una sola respuesta)*

    ☐ Sólo los hombres
    ☐ Por la mayor parte, los hombres
    ☐ Tanto los hombres como las mujeres
    ☐ Por la mayor parte, las mujeres
    ☐ Sólo las mujeres
    ☐ No sé

17. Usted se considera: *(Por favor seleccione una sola respuesta)*

    ☐ Heterosexual
    ☐ Homosexual
    ☐ Bisexual
    ☐ Otro *(por favor especifique)* _____
    ☐ No sé

---

En el resto de las preguntas de este cuestionario, vamos a preguntarle acerca de sexo oral, anal y vaginal. Por favor, sírvase ver las definiciones a continuación.

> *Sexo oral = contacto de la boca con la vagina, el pene, o el ano*
> *Sexo anal = inserción del pene en el ano*
> *Sexo vaginal = inserción del pene en la vagina*

---

18. En los últimos 3 meses, ha tenido relaciones sexuales (por vía vaginal, oral, o anal) ya sea con hombres o con mujeres? *(Por favor seleccione una sola respuesta)*

    ☐ Sí
    ☐ No *(Si responde "No", por favor pase a la pregunta No. 26)*

19. En los últimos 3 meses, ¿cuántas parejas sexuales ha tenido? *(Por favor seleccione una sola respuesta)*

    ☐ 1        ☐ 5–10
    ☐ 2        ☐ 11–20
    ☐ 3        ☐ 21–50
    ☐ 4        ☐ 51 o más

20. En los últimos 3 meses, ¿ha intercambiado relaciones sexuales por dinero, drogas, u otros productos o servicios?

    ☐ Sí
    ☐ No

21. En los últimos 3 meses, ¿cuántas veces ha tenido relaciones sexuales cuando usted o su pareja sexual estaba bajo el efecto de alcohol o drogas (como por ejemplo marihuana, cocaína, heroína o crack)?

    _____ veces *(indique el número de veces)*

22. En los últimos 3 meses, ¿cuántos compañeros (solamente MASCULINOS) de relaciones sexuales ha tenido?

    _____ *(Indique el número de compañeros masculinos)*
    *(Si la respuesta a compañeros masculinos es 0, pase a la pregunta No. 24)*

**23.** Por favor marque con un círculo el número que indique las veces que <u>en los últimos 3 meses</u>, ha realizado cada una de las siguientes actividades con su/s compañero/s de relaciones sexuales <u>MASCULINO/S</u>:

*(Si Ud. es un hombre, por favor salte la pregunta "a" acerca de las relaciones sexuales pene-vaginales)*

| | No he hecho esta actividad sexual <u>en los últimos 3 meses</u> | 0 veces | 1–5 veces | 6–10 veces | 11–20 veces | 21–50 veces | 51+ veces |
|---|---|---|---|---|---|---|---|
| a. Relación sexual pene-vaginal sin usar condón | 1 | 2 | 3 | 4 | 5 | 6 | 7 |
| b. Relación sexual pene-anal sin usar condón | 1 | 2 | 3 | 4 | 5 | 6 | 7 |
| c. Sexo por vía oral (usted lo hacía a su compañero) sin usar condón, protección dental o protección de plástico que no va al microondas | 1 | 2 | 3 | 4 | 5 | 6 | 7 |

**24.** <u>En los últimos 3 meses</u> cuántas compañeras (<u>solamente FEMENINAS</u>) de relaciones sexuales ha tenido?
_____ *(Indique el número de compañeras)*
*(Si la respuesta al número de compañeras es 0, pase a la pregunta No. 26)*

**25.** Por favor marque con un círculo el número que indique las veces que en <u>los últimos 3 meses</u> ha realidado cada una de las siguientes actividades con su/s compañera/s de relaciones sexuales <u>FEMENINA/S</u>:

*(Si Ud. es una mujer, por favor salte la pregunta "a" acerca de las relaciones sexuales pene-vaginales y la pregunta "b" acerca de relaciones sexuales pene-anales)*

| | No he hecho esta actividad sexual <u>en los últimos 3 meses</u> | 0 veces | 1–5 veces | 6–10 veces | 11–20 veces | 21–50 veces | 51+ veces |
|---|---|---|---|---|---|---|---|
| a. Relación sexual pene-vaginal sin usar condón | 1 | 2 | 3 | 4 | 5 | 6 | 7 |
| b. Relación sexual pene-anal sin usar condón | 1 | 2 | 3 | 4 | 5 | 6 | 7 |
| c. Sexo por vía oral (usted lo hacía a su compañera) sin usar condón, protección dental o protección de plástico que no va al microondas | 1 | 2 | 3 | 4 | 5 | 6 | 7 |

**26.** ¿Es usted hispano/a o latino/a? *(Por favor seleccione solo una respuesta)*
☐ Sí
☐ No

**27.** La mayoría de las personas se consideran miembros de un grupo racial determinado. ¿Con cuál(es) de las categorías siguientes se identifica Ud.?
☐ Blanco/a
☐ Nativo/a de Alaska
☐ Nativo/a de Hawai

☐ Indígena
☐ Afro-Americano/a
☐ Otro Negro/a
☐ Asiático/a
☐ Isleño/a del Pacífico
☐ Raza Mezclada *(por favor especifique)* _____
☐ Otro *(por favor especifique)* _____

**28. Para cada una de las actividades siguientes, por favor indique con qué idioma(s) se siente más cómodo/a:**

| | Sólo inglés | Inglés por la mayor parte | Inglés y otro/s idioma/s por igual | Otro/s idioma/s por la mayor parte | Sólo otro/s idioma/s |
|---|---|---|---|---|---|
| a. Hablar con amigos íntimos | 1 | 2 | 3 | 4 | 5 |
| b. Hablar con la familia en casa | 1 | 2 | 3 | 4 | 5 |
| c. Leer libros, revistas, periódicos | 1 | 2 | 3 | 4 | 5 |
| d. Escuchar la radio | 1 | 2 | 3 | 4 | 5 |

**29. Si usa otro(s) idioma(s) a pesar del inglés y el español, por favor indique qué idioma/s usa:** _____

**HA LLEGADO AL FINAL DEL CUESTIONARIO.**
***MUCHAS GRACIAS* POR HABERLO COMPLETADO.**

# Tool 4-17 Software and Online Tools

A number of computer-based data analysis tools that may be helpful for your outcome evaluation efforts are listed below.

**Popular Statistical Analysis Programs**
- MS Excel: http://office.microsoft.com/home/office.aspx?assetid=FX01085800.aspx
- SPSS: http://www.spss.com/
- SAS: http://www.sas.com/index.html

**Popular Qualitative Analysis Software**
- Ethnograph: http://www.QualisResearch.com
- NVivo, N6, and XSight: http://www.qsrinternational.com/products/productoverview/product_overview.htm

**Online Survey Creation, Data Collection, and Analysis**
- From the Centers for Disease Control and Prevention (CDC): http://www.cdcnpin.org/scripts/tools/software.asp
  - Epi-Info (quantitative analysis)
  - CDC EZ-Text (qualitative analysis)
  - AnSWR (to integrate quantitative/qualitative analysis)
- Survey Monkey: http://www.surveymonkey.com/
- From Sociometrics Corporation:
  - Virtual Program Evaluation Consultant (VPEC) for HIV/AIDS Prevention Programs: http://www.socio.com/vpec/

## Tool 4-18 Matrix for Disseminating Your Findings[1]

It is important to think through how you will disseminate the findings of your outcome evaluation to key audiences. The matrix below will help you do this.

To fill in the worksheet on your computer (using the file on the CD-ROM), click on the gray-shaded area in the box you would like to type in. (Note that the gray shading will not appear in printouts of this document.)

| Audience | Methods for Sharing Results, e.g.:<br>■ *Report*<br>■ *Report summary*<br>■ *Fact sheet*<br>■ *Newsletter article*<br>■ *Newspaper article*<br>■ *Web page or agency Web site*<br>■ *Meeting or event presentation*<br>■ *Radio interview* | Who Will Take the Lead | Timeframe |
|---|---|---|---|
| **Colleagues at Your Agency** | | | |
| **Board of Directors** | | | |
| **Colleagues at Other Agencies** | | | |
| **Clients** | | | |
| **Other Community Members** | | | |
| **Policy Makers** | | | |
| **Funders** | | | |
| **Other** *(specify:)* | | | |

[1] Adapted from Card, J. J., Brindis, C., Peterson, J. L., & Niego, S. (2001). *Guidebook: Evaluating teen pregnancy prevention programs* (2nd ed., Exercise 4.5). Los Altos, CA: Sociometrics Corporation.

# Glossary

## A

**ad hoc interpreter**—An ad hoc interpreter is a person (such as an agency administrative assistant or a client's friend or relative) whose primary job function is something other than interpretation. An ad hoc interpreter should be used in a service encounter only when neither an appropriately trained bilingual service staff member nor a *professional interpreter* is available. (See also *interpreter.*)

**adaptation**—Adaptation is a process of altering something (e.g., program, policy, or evaluation instrument) to reduce mismatches between its characteristics and the new context in which is it to be implemented or used. Appropriate adaptation requires a thorough understanding of the original program, policy, or instrument and the differences between the original and new target population, community context, and implementing agency or group.

**AIDS Risk Reduction Model**—This model uses elements of several other models (including the *Diffusion of Innovations Theory, Health Belief Model, Social Cognitive Theory,* and others) to organize behavior change factors specific to HIV risk reduction. It is a stage model comprising three behavioral change steps: (1) recognition of HIV infection risk; (2) commitment to behavior change, which may include changes in attitudes and self-efficacy; and (3) enactment of behavior change, which may include gaining support from others, communicating with others about change, and initiating change.

**analysis**—Analysis involves taking a systematic approach to a problem. This includes simplifying the problem into its constitutive parts; identifying facts, assumptions, and purposes of the problem; and formulating a conclusion regarding the problem.

**anonymity**—Anonymity is a state in which a person's individual identity or personal identifying information is unknown to others and cannot be discovered. By not disclosing identifiable characteristics or information (e.g., appearance, Social Security number, date of birth, etc), a person's identity remains unspecified. An anonymous survey does not collect or include any information that can potentially link survey responses to the individual from whom they are obtained. (See also *confidentiality.*)

**assent**—Assent is a term that is often used to refer to the voluntary agreement by a minor (i.e., defined in most U.S. states as a person under age 18) to participate in a research (including evaluation) study. In addition to minor assent, the *consent* of a parent or legal guardian is usually required for such participation.

**attrition**—Attrition refers to the loss of program or evaluation participants or staff over time. Attrition can threaten the success of a program and the validity of its evaluation, so program and evaluation planners should consider strategies for keeping attrition rates low.

# B

**baseline data**—Outcome-related information gathered from or about study participants prior to program start or exposure is known as baseline data (or *pretest data*). Baseline data are usually compared to data collected during or after program implementation or participation (see *posttest data*). Surveys, intake interviews, and medical record review are some common ways to collect this data.

**behavioral and social science theories** (also called **formal theories**)—Behavioral and social science theories comprise assumptions, principles, and methods about learning, social relationships, and behavior that have already proven useful in explaining behavior or in designing effective interventions in health or social areas. Some examples of general formal theories that form the basis of effective HIV prevention programs include the *Diffusion of Innovations Theory, Harm Reduction Model, Health Belief Model, Social Cognitive Theory, Stages of Change Model (Transtheoretical Model), Theory of Gender and Power,* and *Theory of Reasoned Action.* Examples of theories that are specific to HIV prevention are the *AIDS Risk Reduction Model* and *Information-Motivation-Behavioral Skills (IMB) Model.*

# C

**closed-ended questions**—These are survey or interview questions that require respondents to choose among fixed answer categories (e.g., true/false, multiple choice). (See also *open-ended questions*.)

**collectivism**—Collectivism describes a theoretical or practical emphasis on the group, as opposed to the individual. Societies and groups can differ in the extent to which they are based on "self-regarding" (i.e., individualistic and self-interested) behavior versus "other-regarding" (i.e., group-oriented and group- or society-minded) behavior. A collectivist society is one that sets it priorities based mainly on the needs of the group or larger community and emphasizes the interdependence of group members. (See also *individualism.*)

**community**—A community is a group of persons defined by a common set of characteristics, such as shared location, history, cultural affiliation, values, experiences, occupation, or interest in particular issues or activities. A community can also be a geographic area, such as a census tract, neighborhood, or street.

**community leader**—A community leader can be anyone who is identified by members of a group as a their representative or as someone they respect.

**comparison group**—A comparison group is a group of study participants who are assigned to receive either an alternate intervention to the program being evaluated or no intervention. A comparison group should be maximally similar to the *treatment group* (i.e., the group receiving the intervention being evaluated) on key demographic and personal variables. Inclusion of an appropriate comparison group in an outcome evaluation study increases the potential to determine whether it was the intervention or some other factor (e.g., another program, a policy change, a broader change in societal norms, or maturation) that led to changes observed in the treatment group. When a comparison group is formed through *random* *assignment* of study participants to treatment and comparison groups, it is called a *control group.*

**confidentiality**—Confidentiality refers to keeping private the information that individuals provide under the condition that it not be disclosed without their permission. In research studies, confidentiality most often refers to keeping private any information that could lead to the identification of a research subject. A confidential survey process, for example, may include collection of data or other information (such as name or date of birth) that can potentially be linked to the individual from whom survey responses are obtained. When personal identifying information is collected, however, it is removed from the dataset before publication or presentation of findings. If a key linking a survey code number to this information exists, researchers also keep the key separate from the data, often in a locked facility with limited access. (See also *anonymity* and *privacy.*)

**consent**—See *informed consent.*

**control group**—A control group is a *comparison group* that is formed through *random assignment* of study participants either to receive the intervention being evaluated or to receive an alternate intervention (or no intervention). Inclusion of a control group in an outcome evaluation study increases the potential to determine whether it was the intervention or some other factor (e.g., another program, a policy change, a broader change in societal norms, or maturation) that led to changes observed in the treatment group. Random assignment of study participants to treatment and control groups is often considered to be the "gold standard" in evaluation research, but it is not always the most appropriate or culturally competent design for a particular evaluation study. (See also *experimental design.*)

**core program**—For programs that have demonstrated positive effects on their clients, the core program may be defined as those content and design elements that are responsible for the effectiveness. These elements can be identified based on the *behavioral and social science theories* that underlie the intervention; the experience of the original program developer or evaluator with the program; or research studies that test the effects of different versions of the program (i.e., with and without certain features or elements).

**cultural competence**—Cultural competence may be defined as a set of congruent behaviors, attitudes, and policies—including a consideration for linguistic, socioeconomic, and functional concerns that influence behavior—that come together in a system, agency, or among professionals, thus: (1) enabling that system, agency, or those professionals to work effectively with the target population and (2) resulting in services that are accepted by the target population.

**culturally competent program implementation**—Culturally competent HIV prevention program implementation involves community leaders in program activities, monitors ongoing and emerging target population needs, makes appropriate midcourse program adjustments to meet these needs, addresses barriers to effective communication, encourages staff and participant feedback, and respects cultural diversity. (See also *cultural competence; program implementation.*)

**culturally competent program planning**—Culturally competent HIV prevention program planning includes a "look inward" at staff and agency norms, values, and assumptions; involves the target community actively in the planning process; considers the linguistic, socioeconomic, and other cultural factors that influence HIV risk behaviors; and strives to create services that are appropriate for and accepted by the target population. (See also *cultural competence; program planning.*)

**culturally competent program evaluation**—Culturally competent HIV prevention program evaluation involves incorporating awareness of the cultural norms, attitudes, and beliefs of the communities your program serves into all aspects of the evaluation. Involving program stakeholders (staff, community members, and representatives of the program's target population) in all evaluation activities, from design to data collection, analysis, interpretation, and reporting, can help ensure that this happens. (See also *cultural competence; program evaluation.*)

**culture**—Cultures comprise widely shared sets of values, institutions, practices, and beliefs that emerge and change as groups adapt to their environment. Culture is learned through social interactions that provide contexts for behavior and influence behavior.

# D

**data**—Data constitute a collection of information that allows a researcher or evaluator to address one or more questions or interest.

**data cleaning**—Data cleaning is the process of identifying and correcting *data coding* or data entry errors.

**data coding**—Data coding is the process of assigning each piece of data (such as a respondent's answer to a survey or interview question) a specific code or value so that the data can be analyzed in a systematic way.

**dedicated interpreter**—See *professional interpreter*.

**Diffusion of Innovations Theory**—This theory addresses how ideas, products, and practices that are new (or perceived as new) spread within an organization or community, or from one society to another.

**dissemination**—Dissemination refers to those activities that publicize or distribute information about the content, format, processes, or outcomes of a program or project, in order to inform others of the findings, promote policy development, or promote replication of the program or project. Examples of strategies for disseminating evaluation results include presentations to agency boards, funders, staff, community members, and colleagues; articles in journals, newsletters, magazines, newspapers, or on Web sites; and press conferences.

# E

**ethnography**—Ethnography is a qualitative research method that seeks to identify and describe in careful detail and sufficient depth the particular sociocultural practices of a group, organization, institution, community, or system through immersion in its customs, practices, and beliefs. The researcher seeks a comprehensive portrait and understanding of individual and collective views. Ethnography often involves long-term observation of and interaction with persons or groups in their own context, without any attempt to manipulate their environment for research purposes. It is particularly useful for identifying specific, locally based views, beliefs, constructions, and ideas.

**evaluation**—In social, behavioral, educational, and public health research, evaluation refers to the systematic analysis of a program or policy to determine what it has provided or offered, for whom, how, and with what effects. It often focuses specifically on whether a program has delivered the services it intended to deliver, reached the population it intended to reach, and achieved the desired *objectives* and *goals* with respect to the target population.

**experimental design**—An outcome evaluation with an experimental design uses *random assignment* to assign participants to a *treatment group* (which receives the intervention being evaluated) and a *control group* (which receives either no intervention or an alternate intervention). It is often considered the "gold standard" in evaluation design, but it is not necessarily the most appropriate or culturally competent design for a given target population, community, and agency context.

**external evaluator**—An external evaluator (or *outside evaluator*) is an evaluation lead who comes from outside the agency that is conducting the program or project that is being evaluated. An external evaluator can bring a helpful outside perspective and increased credibility to an evaluation study. He or she should work closely with key program stakeholders to ensure that the evaluation is conducted in a culturally competent manner and that the findings are useful to all stakeholder groups.

**external validity**—If the results of a study can be generalized to other circumstances beyond those of the specific context in which the study was conducted, they are considered to be externally valid. (See also *internal validity, validity.*)

# F

**field research**—Anthropological, social, or behavioral research that observes individuals or groups in their own environment, without intervening in or manipulating their surroundings or common routines, is referred to as field research.

**focus group**—A focus group is a small discussion group led by a trained facilitator for the purpose of collecting information about the target population's attitudes or beliefs on a specific topic. Focus groups can be useful methods for collecting needs and assets assessment data and some types of evaluation data (particularly data on client or staff satisfaction with a program).

**follow-up data**—See *posttest data.*

**formal theories** (or **formal behavioral theories**)—See *behavioral and social science theories.*

**formative evaluation**—A formative evaluation takes place in the early (or formative) stages of a program and is used to revise and strengthen program goals, objectives, and strategies. Formative evaluations generally include *process evaluation* activities and may include basic *outcome evaluation* activities as well.

# G

**goals**—Goals are the long-term changes or states that a program (or policy) seeks to achieve in a target population or target entity. In HIV prevention, these generally focus on HIV-related behaviors and health status (such as STI status or HIV *serostatus*).

# H

**HAART**—HARRT is the abbreviation for "highly active antiretroviral therapy." HAART was introduced in 1996 as a treatment for HIV infection. It uses a combination of several drugs that inhibit the ability of the HIV virus to multiply in the body, thus slowing down the development of AIDS. Use of HAART has contributed to a decline in the annual AIDS death rates in the United States.

**Harm Reduction Model**—This approach does not seek to eliminate or reduce harmful or risky behaviors, but instead focuses on ways to prevent the negative consequences of these behaviors, based on current attitudes and beliefs.

**Health Belief Model**—According to this model, a person takes action (or does not take action) to prevent or treat an illness based on such factors as perception of the existence of a health threat, the benefits of avoiding the threat, environmental cues, and confidence in his or her ability to take action.

**human subjects**—Researchers (including evaluators) observe the physiological or behavioral characteristics of individuals in response to some intervention for the purposes of investigation and analysis. Federal regulations define human subjects as individuals from whom researchers collect data through intervention or interaction, or whose medical or program-related information they analyze.

# I

**impacts**—See *outcomes*.

**individualism**—Individualism describes a theoretical or practical emphasis on the individual, as opposed to the group. Societies and groups can differ in the extent to which they are based upon "self-regarding" (i.e., individualistic and self-interested) behavior versus "other-regarding" (i.e., group-oriented and group- or society-minded) behavior. An individualist society is one that sets it priorities based primarily on the needs of the individual and emphasizes self-reliance and personal independence. (See also *collectivism*.)

**Information-Motivation-Behavioral Skills (IMB) Model**—This model is based on the assumption that information about HIV risk reduction and motivation to reduce HIV risk influence each other and are necessary to develop HIV risk-reduction skills, and that information, motivation, and skills are all crucial to reducing HIV risk behavior.

**informed consent**—Informed consent refers to voluntary agreement by an individual to participate in a research (including evaluation) study after he or she has been provided with detailed information about the study and been equipped with an understanding of study content, procedures, and potential benefits and risks for participants and others. It can also refer to similar voluntary agreement by a parent or legal guardian for his/her minor child to participate in a study. (See also *assent*.)

**Institutional Review Board (IRB)**—An IRB is a group of qualified researchers versed in human subjects protection issues who review research (including evaluation) designs and methods. Their job is to ensure that the designs and methods sufficiently protect the well-being of subjects who will participate in the research and any others who may be affected by the research.

**interpreter**—An interpreter is a practitioner of interpreting, an activity that consists of establishing oral or gestural communication between two or more persons who are not speaking (or signing) the same language. A *translator* is distinguished from an interpreter by the translator's focus on written texts instead of spoken or gestural (signed) language.

**internal validity**—Internal validity refers to the degree to which study findings accurately represent the causal relationship between an intervention and the observed changes or outcomes among participants who have received it. (See also *external validity, validity.*)

**intervention group**—See *treatment group.*

# L

**linguistically isolated**—The U.S. Census considers a person to be "linguistically isolated" if he or she lives in a household in which no member age 14 or over self-identifies as speaking English "very well."

**logic model**—See *program model.*

**logistical barriers (to program participation)**—Logistical barriers are physical impediments to program participation, such as inaccessible times or locations, fees that clients cannot afford, or lack of staff who speak clients' languages.

**long-term goals**—See *goals.*

# M

**mid-term objectives**—See *objectives.*

# N

**needs and assets assessment**—Needs and assets assessment can be defined as the process of collecting and assessing data that describe the nature and magnitude of a community's needs, as well as its resources or assets (e.g., financial, organizational, intellectual, institutional, and human).

# O

**objectives**—Objectives are the short-term or mid-term changes or states that a program (or policy) seeks to achieve in a target population or target entity. In HIV prevention, these generally focus on HIV-related knowledge, attitudes, beliefs, intentions, skills, and behaviors.

**open-ended questions**—These are survey or interview questions that allow respondents to reply using their own words, rather than choosing among fixed answer categories. Open-ended questions produce qualitative data that can be thematically coded by the researcher or evaluator. (See also *close-ended questions.*)

**opinion leader**—An opinion leader is a member of a community whose views or opinions are respected by other community members.

**outcome evaluation**—An outcome evaluation examines whether a program (or policy) actually achieved the desired changes or states (e.g., with respect to knowledge, attitudes, skills, intentions, behaviors, health status, etc.) among the target population.

**outcomes**—Outcomes refer to that which happens to individuals, groups, or populations as the result of an intervention. For example, health outcomes refer to the health status (e.g., the HIV *serostatus*) of individuals, groups, or populations that results from a planned intervention (or series of interventions). Outcomes can also refer to changes in organizations, systems, or policies. Long-term outcomes are sometimes referred to as *impacts*.

**outside evaluator**—See *external evaluator.*

# P

**perceived barriers (to program participation)**—Perceived barriers are psychological impediments to program participation, such as discomfort with program staff, concern about loss of confidentiality, embarrassment about discussing sensitive topics, and fear of arrest or deportation.

**policy**—A policy is a plan of action or process pursued by an individual or institution to achieve a specific end with maximal effectiveness and efficiency. It generally involves the articulation of specific programs and/or procedures and how to apply them concretely. Policy may also refer to sets of rules, as established by laws or internal regulations, that guide organizations.

**posttest data**—Outcome-related information gathered from or about study participants during or after program exposure is known as posttest data. Posttest data are usually compared to data collected before program implementation or participation (see *pretest data*). Posttest data collected after a period of months or years have elapsed since the completion of program implementation are sometimes called *follow-up data.* Surveys, interviews, and medical record review are some common ways to collect this data.

**pretest data**—Outcome-related information gathered from or about study participants before program start or exposure is known as pretest data (or *baseline data*). Baseline data are usually compared to data collected during program or after program implementation or participation (see *posttest data*). Surveys, intake interviews, and medical record review are some common ways to collect this data.

**privacy**—Privacy refers to individuals' ability to keep personal information (e.g., physical, behavioral, emotional, intellectual, political, or demographic) to themselves and to determine whether, how, and with whom it will be shared. In a research or evaluation study, privacy is maintained when study participants or researchers/evaluators prevent others from accessing this information, unless the individuals themselves choose to make it public.

**problem statement**—A problem statement offers a synopsis of the issues, problems, and needs facing a community, as well as the resources and strategies that might address these needs. It provides the perspective needed for subsequent program planning tasks, such as setting *goals* and *objectives* and planning *program components*.

**process evaluation**—A process evaluation assesses the program as implemented versus what was planned. As such, it can document whether the intended activities or services were delivered, whether the intended target population was reached, and whether the intended resources were used. Process evaluation can also include assessment of participant and staff satisfaction of the program as delivered.

**professional interpreter**—A professional interpreter (or *dedicated interpreter*) is an individual whose sole function in the service setting is to interpret. (See also *interpreter* and *ad hoc interpreter.*)

**program components**—Program components are the prevention activities or services that will be used or offered to achieve specified objectives and goals for a particular population. For each component, the prevention approach, content, delivery format, duration and frequency, implementation setting, and staffing can be specified.

**program evaluation**—Program evaluation refers to the systematic assessment of a program, including such questions as whether and how it delivered the intended services, reached the intended population, or achieved the desired outcomes.

**program implementation**—Program implementation refers to the provision of program activities or services to clients or to a population. It also includes a number of related tasks that must be carried out concurrently to keep the program running, such as recruiting and retaining program participants, retaining staff, and managing the program (e.g., overseeing staff, tracking expenditures, etc.).

**program model**—A program model (or *logic model*) is a visual representation of a program's goals and objectives, and the program components that link to them. A program model provides a visual overview of the program's *theory of change.*

**program planning**—Program planning encompasses a wide range of research, strategizing, networking, and coordinating activities that—if done well—lay the groundwork for successful program implementation and assessment. Program activities may include (but are not limited to): identifying community *needs and assets;* defining the *target population* and the problem/issue that the program will address; identifying program *goals* and *objectives;* defining *program components;* developing a *program model;* making decisions about whether to *replicate* an existing program or develop a new program; recruiting and training staff; and planning for *evaluation.*

**protocol**—A protocol is the design or plan for a specific research activity. It describes the research approach and methodology, eligibility requirements for study participants, the treatment or intervention that will occur (and any comparison or control conditions that will be included), and data analysis procedures. It can also refer to an individual data collection instrument, such as a survey or a question guide for a focus group or interview.

**protocol analysis**—This is a procedure that can help reveal problems with the wording or approach of data collection instruments such as surveys, interview questions, or focus group question guides. Individuals or small groups review the instrument in the presence of a researcher or evaluator and are encouraged to "think aloud" as they formulate a response to each question. A series of follow-up questions about the instrument may also be asked.

# Q

**quasi-experimental design**—A quasi-experimental design is an outcome evaluation design that includes a *treatment group,* which participates in the intervention being evaluated, and a well-matched (but not *randomly assigned*) *comparison group,* which receives either a different intervention or no intervention.

# R

**random assignment**—In an outcome evaluation with an *experimental design,* each study participant has an equal chance of being assigned to the *treatment group* (which receives the intervention being evaluated) or the *control group* (which receives an alternate or no intervention), because this assignment is random, or based on chance. Random assignment increases the likelihood that differences observed between treatment and control groups are the result of the intervention being evaluated, and not some other intervening factor or variable that has different effects on the two groups. Random assignment of study participants to treatment and control groups is often considered to be the "gold standard" in evaluation research, but it is not always the most appropriate or culturally competent design for a particular evaluation study.

**recruitment**—Recruitment refers to locating, earning the trust of, and enrolling members of the target audience in an HIV prevention program. It may also refer to locating and offering positions to appropriate paid or volunteer staff members.

**reliability**—In research, reliability concerns the quality or consistency of a measurement or service. The degree to which a test, experiment, or measure produces the same results on repeated application is the degree to which it is reliable. Having high reliability is necessary (but not sufficient) to achieve high *validity.*

**replication**—Replication is the process of moving an intervention to a new site in a way that maintains fidelity (faithfulness) to the *core program* but also permits adaptations to the new context.

**research site**—See *site visit.*

**retention**—Retention refers to the extent to which programs or evaluation studies are able to retain their participants (or staff) over a given period of time.

**risk**—Risk is an important concept for research with human subjects. It refers to the likelihood that some form of harm may befall subjects who participate in a research study. Researchers should always minimize risk to study participants.

# S

**self-efficacy**—Self-efficacy is the belief in one's own ability to perform a behavior in different circumstances.

**semistructured interview**—In a semistructured interview, the interviewee is asked mainly *open-ended questions* and is encouraged to provide detailed responses and examples.

**serostatus**—A person's HIV serostatus is determined by a blood test for antibodies to the Human Immunodeficiency Virus. HIV serostatus is "positive" if the test detects antibodies to HIV. HIV serostatus is "negative" if the test does not detect antibodies to HIV.

**short-term objectives**—See *objectives.*

**site visit**—A site visit for research purposes involves researchers visiting a location at which data will be collected (also known as a *research site*) and collecting this data through methods such as interviews, focus groups, or surveys. Making a site visit is a type of *field research.*

**Social Cognitive Theory**—According to this theory, personal factors (such as skills, motivation, and *self-efficacy* to perform a behavior), environmental factors (particularly modeling and reinforcement of behavior), and behaviors themselves influence each other.

**Social Learning Theory**—This theory was the precursor to *Social Cognitive Theory* and is often used interchangeably with Social Cognitive Theory.

**Stages of Change Model**—This model, also called the *Transtheoretical Model,* describes people's readiness and motivation to change their behavior as a series of stages that range from no intention to change behavior, to thinking about and preparing to change behavior, to enacting and maintaining behavior change.

**staff**—Staff comprise the employees, consultants, interns, and volunteers who carry out work on behalf of an agency, program, or project.

**subjects**—See *human subjects.*

**structured interview or survey**—This is an interview or survey in which the respondent is asked mainly *closed-ended questions* (e.g., true/false, multiple choice), so that responses can easily be compared across individuals and over time.

**survey**—A survey is a set of questions designed to collect readily quantifiable information from a group of individuals, often for health, social science, public opinion, or other research purposes. Surveys can be conducted in writing, over the Internet, by phone, and through face-to-face interactions. Surveys may be completed directly by participants or by researchers who record participants' responses to questions posed in *structured interviews*. Sometimes computers with audio or video capability are used to assist persons with limited literacy skills to complete surveys.

# T

**target population**—A target population is the group of people whom a specific intervention is designed to influence. A clearly defined target population is essential for successful program planning, implementation, and evaluation.

**theory of change**—A theory of change is a theory about how *program components* (i.e., program activities or services) will lead to desired *objectives* and *goals* (i.e., changes or states) in a target population or target entity. (See also *behavioral and social science theories.*)

**Theory of Gender and Power**—This theory examines how certain social structures shape the relationships between men and women and the lives that they lead. These social structures include the sexual division of labor (e.g., how men's versus women's work arrangements shape their lives); the sexual division of power (e.g., the levels of power men and women have in different areas of life, and the consequences of these arrangements); and social norms and social attachments (e.g., society's expectations and beliefs about women and men's behaviors, including sexual behaviors, and how these influence women's and men's lives).

**Theory of Planned Behavior**—According to this theory, which grew out of the *Theory of Reasoned Action*, a person's beliefs, attitudes, and perceived control over a behavior influence behavioral intentions, which in turn influence behaviors.

**Theory of Reasoned Action**—According to this theory, a person's beliefs and attitudes influence behavioral intentions, which in turn influence behaviors. (See also *Theory of Planned Behavior.*)

**translator**—A translator is a practitioner of translation, an activity that consists of determining the meaning of a written text in one language (i.e., the source text) and producing a new, equivalent text in another language (called the target text, or the translation). An *interpreter* is distinguished from a translator by the interpreter's focus on spoken or gestural (signed) language, instead of written language.

**Transtheoretical Model**—See *Stages of Change Model.*

**treatment group**—The treatment group (or *intervention group*) is the group in an evaluation study that receives the intervention that is being evaluated. (See also *comparison group* and *control group.*)

# V

**validity**—Validity refers to the degree to which an instrument, experiment, or other study measures that which it is designed to measure. When results accurately reflect the concept being measured, they can be considered valid.

## REFERENCES

The California Endowment (2005). Glossary. Woodland Hills, CA: The California Endowment. Retrieved November 8, 2005, from http://www.calendow.org/reference/new_glossaryref.stm

Card, J. J., Brindis, C., Peterson, J. L., & Niego, S. (2001). *Guidebook: Evaluating teen pregnancy prevention programs* (2nd ed.). Los Altos, CA: Sociometrics Corporation.

Cross, T. L., Bazron, B. J., Dennis, K. W., & Isaacs, M. R. (1989). *Towards a culturally competent system of care: A monograph on effective services for minority children who are severely emotionally disturbed.* Washington, DC: CASSP Technical Assistance Center, Georgetown University Child Development Center.

Dana, R. H., Behn, J. D. & Gonwa, T. (1992). A checklist for the examination of cultural competence in social service agencies. *Research on Social Work Practice, 2*(2), 220–233.

Herlocher, T., Hoff, C., & DeCarlo, P. (1996). *Can theory help in HIV prevention?* Center for AIDS Prevention Studies (CAPS), University of California San Francisco. Retrieved August 1, 2005, from http://www.hivpositive.com/f-HIVyou/2-Prevention/theorytext.html

Kalichman, S. C. (1998). *Preventing AIDS: A sourcebook for behavioral interventions.* Mahwah, NJ: Lawrence Erlbaum Associates.

Like, R. C., Steiner, R. P., & Rubel, A. J. (1996). STFM core curriculum guidelines: Recommended core curriculum guidelines on culturally sensitive and competent health care. *Family Medicine, 28*(4), 291–297.

National Cancer Institute. (2005). *Theory at a glance: A guide for health promotion practice* (2nd ed.). NIH Publication No. 05–3896. U.S. Department of Health and Human Services, National Institutes of Health. Retrieved May 7, 2006, from http://www.cancer.gov/PDF/481f5d53–63df-41bc-bfaf-5aa48ee1da4d/TAAG3.pdf

Office for Human Research Protections, U.S. Department of Health and Human Services (HHS). (2005). Glossary. *Institutional review board guidebook.* Retrieved September 19, 2005, from http://www.hhs.gov/ohrp/irb/irb_glossary.htm

Shin, H. B., & Bruno, R. (2003). Language use and English-speaking ability: 2000. *Census 2000 Brief, C2KBR-29,* 1–11. Retrieved June 18, 2005, from http://www.census.gov/prod/2003pubs/c2kbr-29.pdf

Vinh-Thomas, P., Bunch, M. M., & Card, J. J. (2003). A research-based tool for identifying and strengthening culturally competent and evaluation-ready HIV/AIDS prevention programs. *AIDS*

*Education and Prevention, 15(6):* 481–98. Retrieved January 16, 2006, from http://www.socio. com/pdf/progarticle2.pdf

Wikipedia, the Free Encyclopedia. [Various entries.] Retrieved August 5, 2005, from http://en. wikipedia.org/wiki/Main_Page

Wingood, G. M., & DiClemente, R. J. (2000). Application of the theory of gender and power to examine HIV-related exposures, risk factors, and effective interventions for women. *Health Education & Behavior, 27*(5), 539–565.

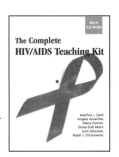

SPRINGER PUBLISHING COMPANY

# Adolescent Sexual Health Education

## *An Activity Sourcebook*

## Josefina Card, PhD, Tabitha Benner, MPA

This useful sourcebook contains more than sixty ready-to-use activities to help practitioners educate teens about pregnancy and STD/HIV/AIDS prevention. The activities are drawn from prevention programs around the country that have been scientifically evaluated and proven to change teens' health behaviors.

The book is divided into six sections based on activity type: role plays, group discussions, homework assignments, group activities, teacher-led discussions, and other modalities. Exercises show teens how to discuss sexual issues and sexuality; how to negotiate condom use; how to protect themselves from STIs/HIV/AIDS; and how to have a greater understanding of gay, lesbian, and bisexual issues.

This wide range of activities can be used by practitioners to develop a sexuality education program from scratch or to supplement an existing program. Most activities can be led by classroom teachers, facilitators, or health educators with no prior experience. The activities are suitable for community-based organizations, health clinics, or classroom settings.

Each activity contains the following information:

- Activity Goal
- Original Program Setting
- Time Needed
- Age Level
- Staff Needed
- Materials Needed (handouts, scripts, etc. are included)
- Activity Description
- Ways to Expand the Activity
- The Original Intervention and Developer

December 2007 · 300 pp (est.) · softcover · 978-0-8261-3822-4

11 West 42nd Street, New York, NY 10036-8002 • Fax: 212-941-7842
Order Toll-Free: 877-687-7476 • Order Online: www.springerpub.com